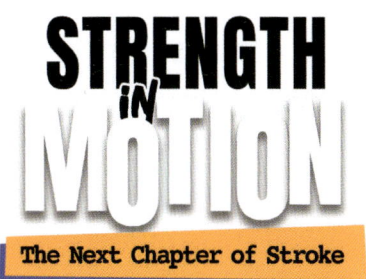

STRENGTH iN MOTION

The Next Chapter of Stroke

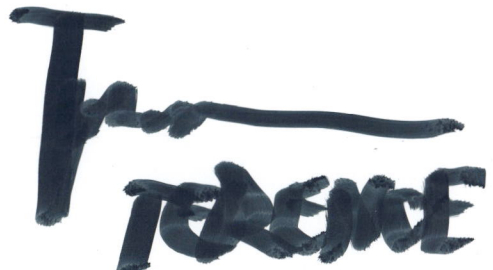

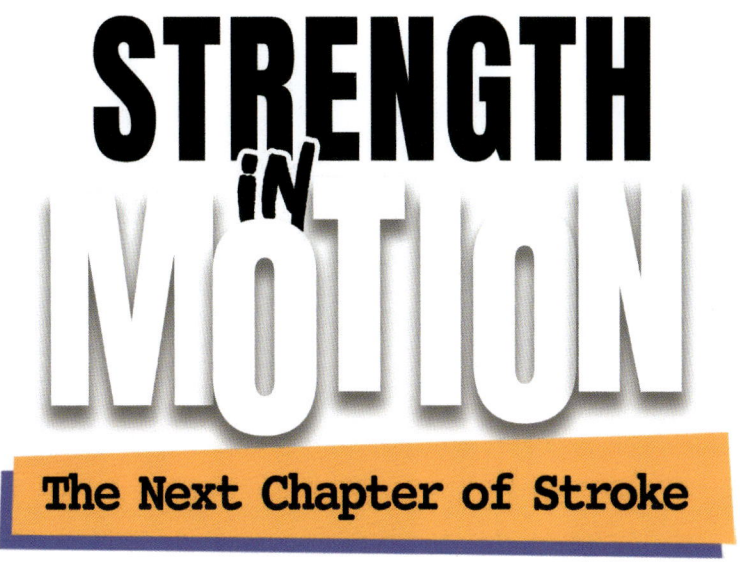

STRENGTH in MOTION

The Next Chapter of Stroke

Terence Ang

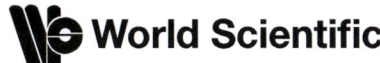

World Scientific

NEW JERSEY · LONDON · SINGAPORE · BEIJING · SHANGHAI · HONG KONG · TAIPEI · CHENNAI · TOKYO

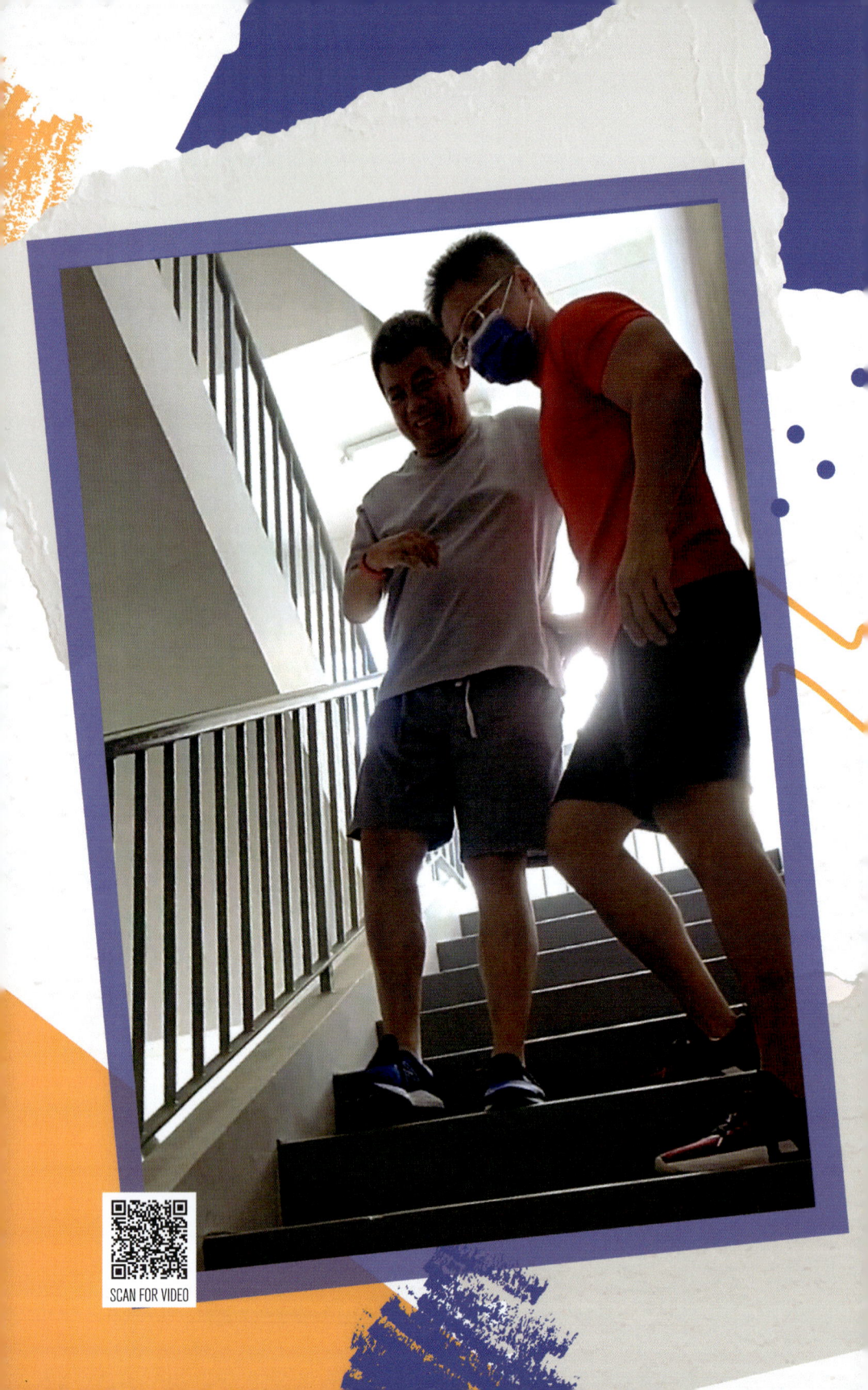

SCAN FOR VIDEO

Strength in Motion: The Next Chapter of Stroke offers a profound look at one man's incredible journey of triumph over adversity, shedding light on the physical, emotional, and psychological hurdles that often characterise the aftermath of a stroke.

From someone gripped by fear to an individual emerging with greater strength and confidence, Terence's story transcends the ordinary and speaks to the indomitable spirit that resides within us all.

Within these pages, readers are taken on a voyage into the transformative power of exercise, witnessing how movement contributes not only to the restoration of physical abilities, but also the reshaping of one's mindset.

The inclusion of medical perspectives and fellow stroke survivors' narratives provide a broader understanding of the complexities inherent in stroke recovery. Complementing the written account are previously unreleased images, a visual diary of Terence's life.

This book aims to empower survivors of stroke, and initiate discussions on how the larger society can offer support and solidarity to those on the path of recovery. The next chapter presents much opportunity to explore innovative approaches, resources, and avenues for enhancing the lives of stroke survivors.

CONTENTS

FOREWORD

I first met Terence at an event commemorating half a century of rehabilitation medicine in Singapore. We struck up a conversation. It was short and took place in the thick of the celebratory cacophony of the anniversary dinner. I left with a sense of unfulfillment because I think there is much more to his life story. I wanted to find out how he thrived in the face of adversity. At least, that is how I see it.

Fortunately, Terence gifted me a copy of his first book, *A Cry in the Dark*. I picked up his book at lunch the next day, thinking that I would read a bit over the ten minutes I had to wolf down my chicken rice before continuing with my Saturday routine. I did not put down the book until I finished it two hours later. I promptly went online and ordered an electronic copy of his second book, *Emerging from the Dark*.

Terence is an individual who refused to acquiesce in the face of a devastating health shock. Stroke is devastating because it not only physically (and sometimes cognitively) cripples the sufferer, it often robs the afflicted of basic functions that one would associate with the dignity of personhood — the ability to be independent in activities of daily living, the empowerment to determine when to do what, the respect for what one is able to achieve, and much more. The abruptness of a stroke event stands in stark contrariety with the long course that the survivor often has to live with its consequences.

Terence's first two books chronicled his medical struggles with stroke, the psychological spirals he experienced, and the breakthroughs he was able to achieve through a combination of positive reframing, relentless determination and the unstinting support of those around him. He narrates his personal journey with fastidious care and a healthy dose of self-deprecating humour, bringing us into the deeper world of a person with stroke. This perspective is often not well appreciated by all except the very survivors themselves.

I am excited about Terence's latest book, *Strength in Motion: The Next Chapter of Stroke*. It offers insights into the plethora of support resources and innovations that can significantly enhance the lives of stroke survivors. Importantly, it demonstrates how modern medical science, technology and complementary therapies, when combined with motivation and will, can improve outcomes for persons with stroke.

We are not yet at the golden age, but what we have today certainly gives hope for optimism. Strokes need not be a disability for life and Terence is the best example.

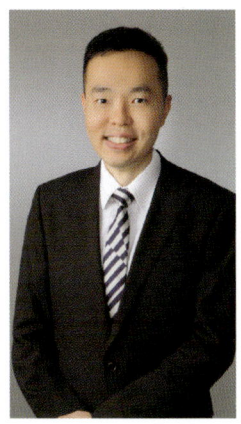

**Associate Professor
Gan Wee Hoe**

*Chief Executive Officer
SingHealth Community Hospitals*

Although rehabilitation medicine is one of 35 recognised specialities in Singapore, it is lesser known than some specialities such as cardiology, neurology, dermatology, etc.

The Australasian Faculty of Rehabilitation Medicine has defined rehabilitation medicine as "the diagnosis, assessment and management of an individual with a disability due to illness or injury. Rehabilitation physicians work with people with a disability to help them achieve an optimal level of performance and improve their quality of life".

Rehabilitation takes a village. It is hard work. As rehabilitation physicians, we work with a multidisciplinary team of nurses and allied health professionals to make up a professional "coaching team" to help patients attain their best potential.

Predicting stroke recovery is not an exact science. Traditional predictors for functional outcome include age, gender, stroke severity, stroke subtype, type of impairments, existing medical conditions, social support, etc. Despite our tools, we cannot predict with absolute certainty. As coaches, we work hand in hand with our patients, striving for the best and preparing for the worst. Patients often surprise us with what they can achieve.

Exercise is medicine. In *Strength in Motion: The Next Chapter of Stroke*, Terence invites us to embark on a profoundly moving journey that transcends the ordinary. His journey vividly illustrates how exercise is more than just a physical endeavour and can reframe one's mindset and stretch the limits of individuals. It is generally safe and perhaps the closest thing we have to a panacea to many chronic medical conditions.

This book serves as a beacon of hope for patients and caregivers grappling with the aftermath of a stroke, and Terence is a source of inspiration for us all. No matter what deck of cards are served to us, only imagine the possibilities.

My patient told me that the commonly used acronym PWD should read as "Persons with Determination" rather than "Persons with

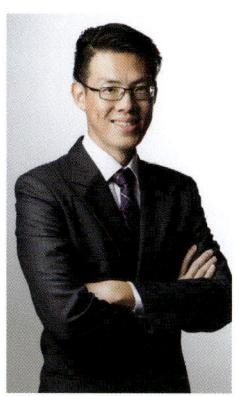

Disabilities". It cannot be more accurate. I look forward to seeing Terence turn more possibilities into realities.

Dr. Wee Tze Chao

MBBS, FAFRM(RACP), FFPMANZCA, FAMS President, Society of Rehabilitation Medicine (Singapore)

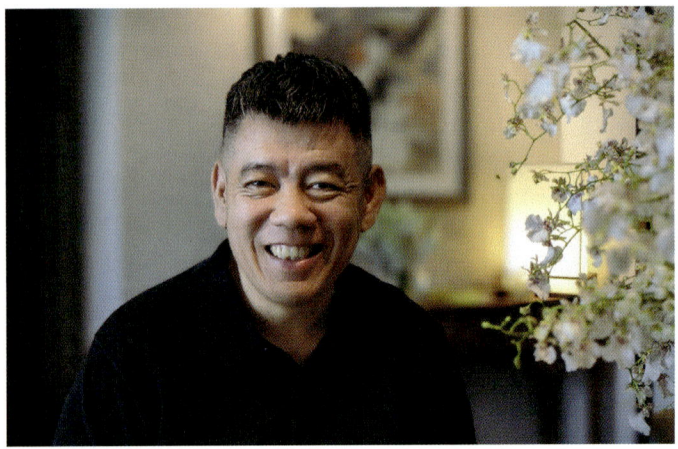

In life, we each navigate our own unique challenges, and my personal journey has been nothing short of a wild ride, a front-row seat to a rollercoaster of twists, turns and loops. Post-stroke recovery has certainly been winding and nonlinear, a long, complex process that continues to test my resilience and spirit.

My first two books, *A Cry in the Dark* and *Emerging from the Dark*, changed my life in many ways. They provided me avenues to process the emotional whirlwind and setbacks I faced during the aftermath of the stroke. At the same

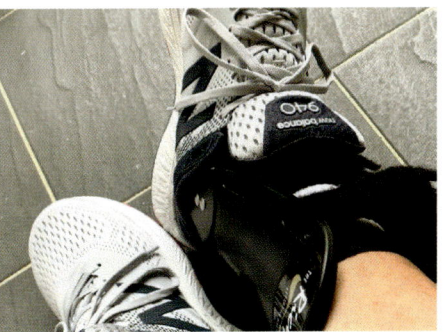

time, they also opened doors I never thought possible. I found myself connecting with fellow stroke survivors, forging bonds over shared experiences and a collective determination to take back control over our lives.

As I moved forward in my story, a new chapter began. A chapter where exercise became my anchor, guiding me toward finding my self-confidence and independence. The freedom to move is one we often overlook, yet it transforms into something truly priceless post-stroke, a fundamental aspect of our daily lives and a key component of our well-being.

This third book grew out of that transformative period, shaped by the shared wisdom of experts, medical professionals, and peers. It is a culmination of the invaluable lessons that have propelled me forward. Through physical effort, I discovered the means to embrace a lively and satisfying life after stroke.

My hope is that those navigating their own storms can find in this book the comfort and motivation to traverse the road ahead. Whether taken with grace or uncertainty, may each step be a reminder that recovery is not a sprint but a steady marathon that unfolds in its own time.

- Terence Ang

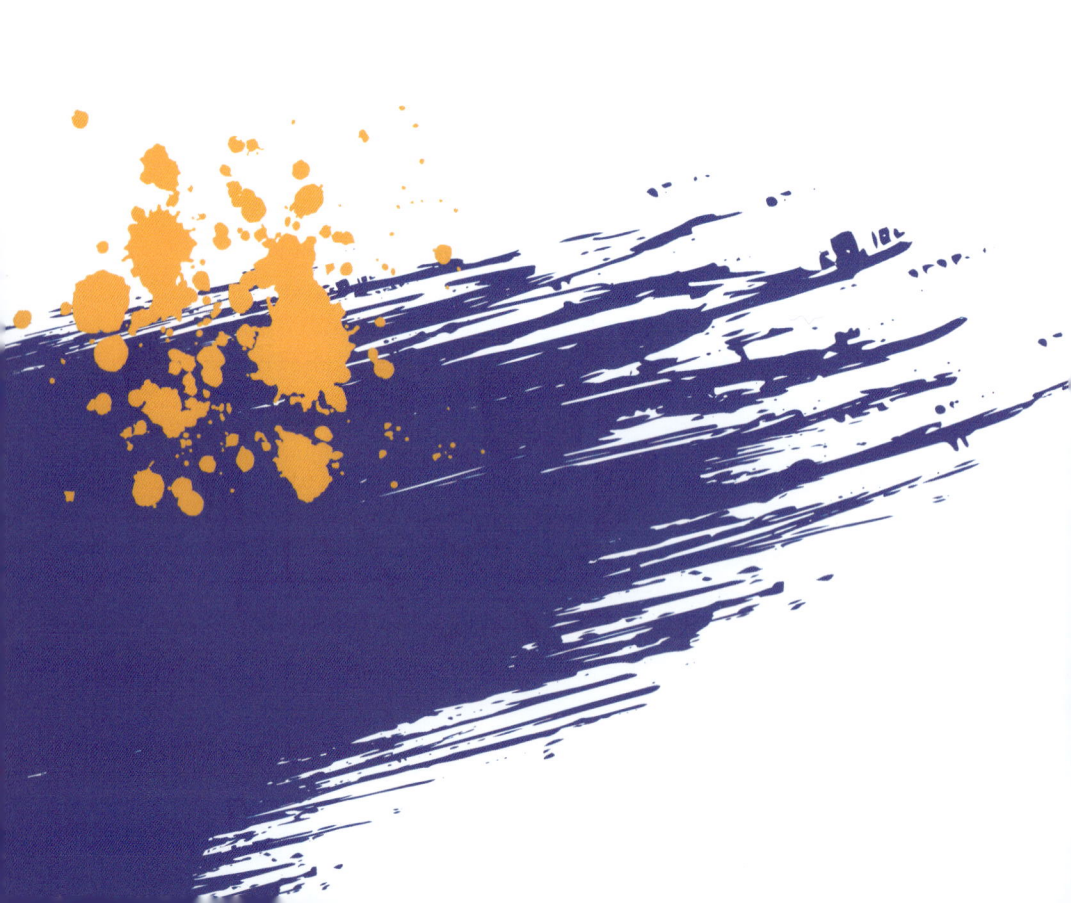

AFTER STROKE... NOW WHAT?

In the sprawling tapestry of our lives, certain events unravel with a startling clarity, forever etching their mark upon the canvas of our existence. For me, such an event was an unexpected wake-up call that would, for better or worse, alter the course of my life.

Stroke. A force that strikes suddenly and without warning. When the storm of a stroke ravages your brain, it leaves a path of destruction and change in its wake. The impact is as unique as the individual it befalls, but no matter the severity or form, one thing is certain. Things will never be the same again.

Grappling with my new reality, I felt a deep sense of anger and resentment within me. Why was I dealt such a cruel hand of misfortune? Why had life chosen this path for me? The questions echoed endlessly in my mind, seeking answers that still remain elusive to me till this day.

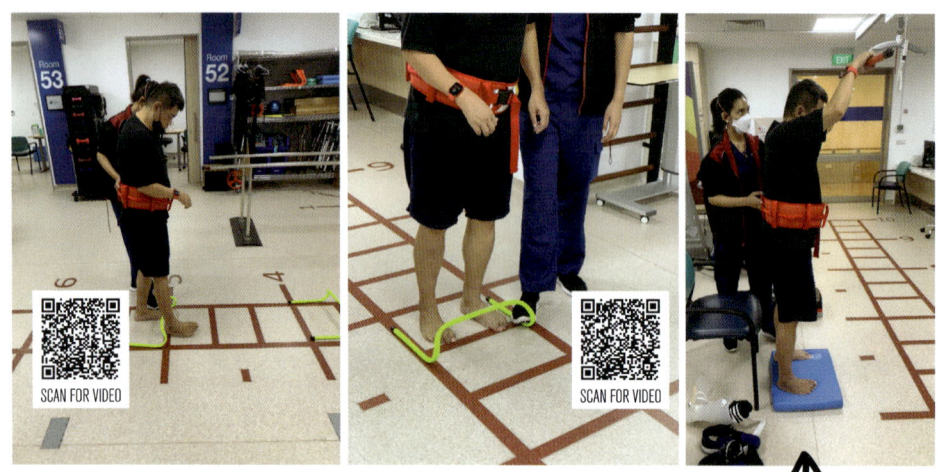

Physical mobility once taken for granted becomes a precious commodity that must be painstakingly regained.

The early days were a slow, torturous climb out of the abyss. I fought tirelessly to regain even the simplest functions — lifting my arm, standing without falling over, or speaking without slurring my words. I spent countless hours in therapy, willing my body to work again.

The frustration of struggling with everyday tasks that had once been second nature cast long shadows over my life. Dependency clung to me like a heavy shroud, a constant reminder of the independence I had lost. I had heard about strokes (and seen stories in the news) but never fully grasped the cruel precision with which it could strip away one's life.

I wanted to feel independent like before unencumbered by anxiety, without the constant reliance on help ...

Simple outings became incredible feats, each one demanding meticulous planning. The idea of venturing outside on my own filled me with trepidation. I needed assistance — a caregiver by my side to bridge the gap between my desires and capabilities. I deeply yearned to move about freely again.

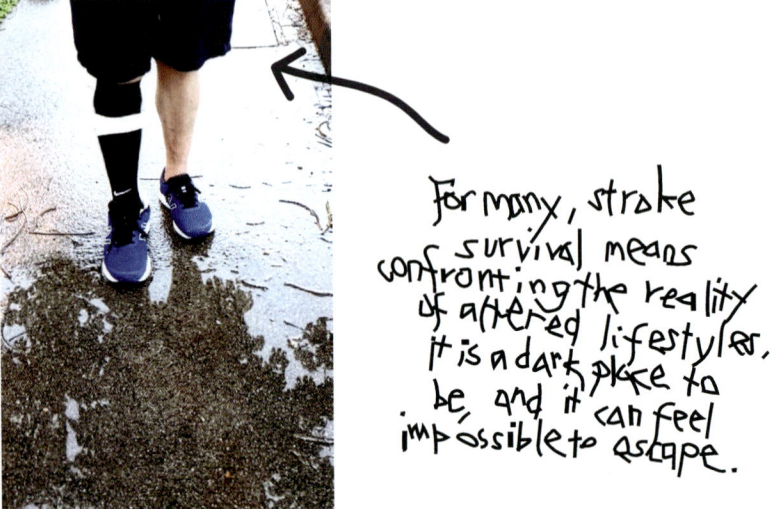

For many, stroke survival means confronting the reality of altered lifestyles. It is a dark place to be, and it can feel impossible to escape.

It is not just our bodies that are affected — our minds, too, bear the scars of the stroke. Cognitive abilities are diminished; memory lapses, difficulty concentrating, and the struggle to find the right words are daily companions. It felt like a constant maze through my own thoughts, and the loss of control was a bitter pill to swallow.

Suddenly, it seemed as if the world around me was mirrored in statistics painting a bleak picture of modern health. The numbers were staggering, a stark reminder that my ordeal was not isolated. The ubiquity of health issues I had often glanced over in reports now came into sharp focus. Stroke, I learned, was not just an affliction of the elderly but a rising epidemic in the 21st century.

It knows no age, gender, or social boundaries. It strikes the young and old alike, with millions affected each year, and both developed as well as developing nations feeling its pervasive reach. And the factors that contribute to this surge in strokes are interwoven into the very fabric of our contemporary lifestyle.

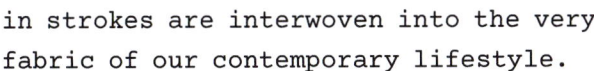

The sedentary existence embraced by many has become a modern-day plague.

Prolonged hours spent seated at desks, commuting in vehicles, or engrossed in screens have shackled us to a life of reduced movement. Poor posture, a subtle consequence of our desk bound jobs, has insidiously invaded our lives. Our bodies were not designed for a life of inertia, yet the modern world demands it.

Although technology has made life easier, physical activity becomes a secondary role, often neglected or pushed to the periphery of our priorities. As the globe hurtles toward a faster pace, our health often takes a backseat, and the consequences are becoming frighteningly apparent.

With the narrative of strokes and broader health issues looming large, it is a persistent reminder of the battles that lie ahead. This has forced me to reflect on my own choices and the fragility of health we often take for granted.

As I began my rehabilitation journey, exercise became a steadfast part of my daily routine. Through perseverance and dedication, I slowly regained not only my physical capabilities but also my sense of self. The first chapter of my new life was unfolding, inscribed with the promise of a healthier tomorrow. And I discovered within motion a transformative power that could rewrite the narrative of strokes.

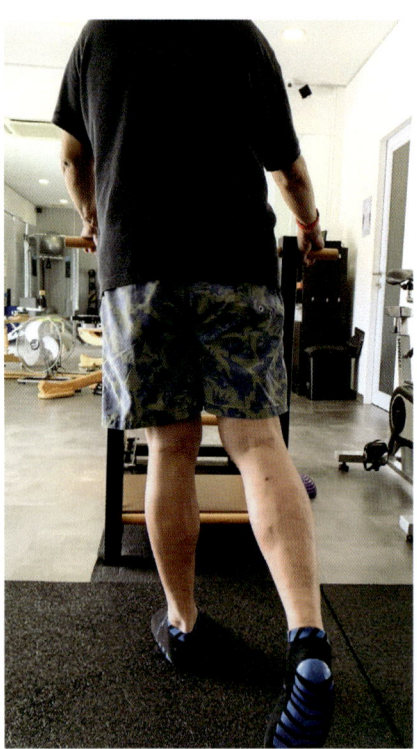

Armed with knowledge and a newfound determination, I refused to be a passive bystander in my life.

Life, in its capricious ways, had presented me with a choice — crumble under the weight of adversity or rise stronger and wiser from its clutches. I shared my story with anyone who would listen, and I found that, like myself, many stroke survivors often face the daunting uncertainty of what lies ahead.

Rebuilding a life after a stroke is a process that extends beyond the immediate challenges of physical therapy. Therapists typically engage with patients during specific phases of rehab, yet they may inadvertently overlook planning for what comes next.

Like when financial constraints limit access to private therapy, pressing questions arise: what awaits such individuals? Can they navigate recovery independently and effectively? Do they possess the requisite self-management skills or know when and how to seek assistance? Are they proactive advocates in their own journey?

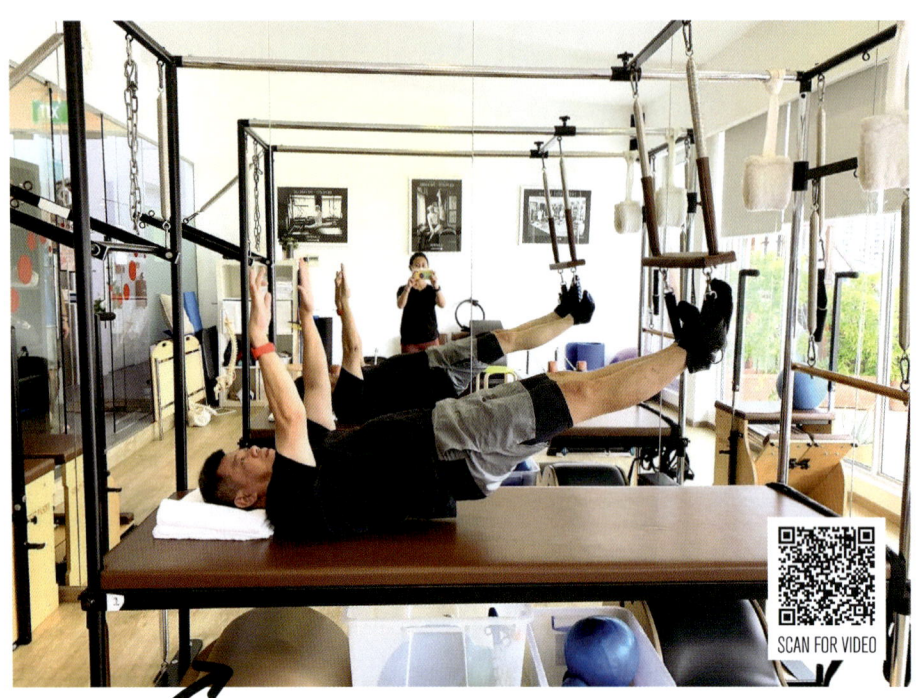

SCAN FOR VIDEO

Within our challenges lie the potential
for growth and healing. It is a call to
redefine our relationship with our
health and well-being.

For those who have experienced the life-altering impact of a stroke, the road ahead can be more than intimidating. But it is important to remember that even in the darkest of times, there is a glimmer of hope.

In this age of breathtaking technological advancements and pioneering medical breakthroughs, we stand at a crossroads. We have a tremendous opportunity to redefine the trajectory of stroke rehabilitation. Recovery is possible, and with the right support and mindset, we can find our way back to the light.

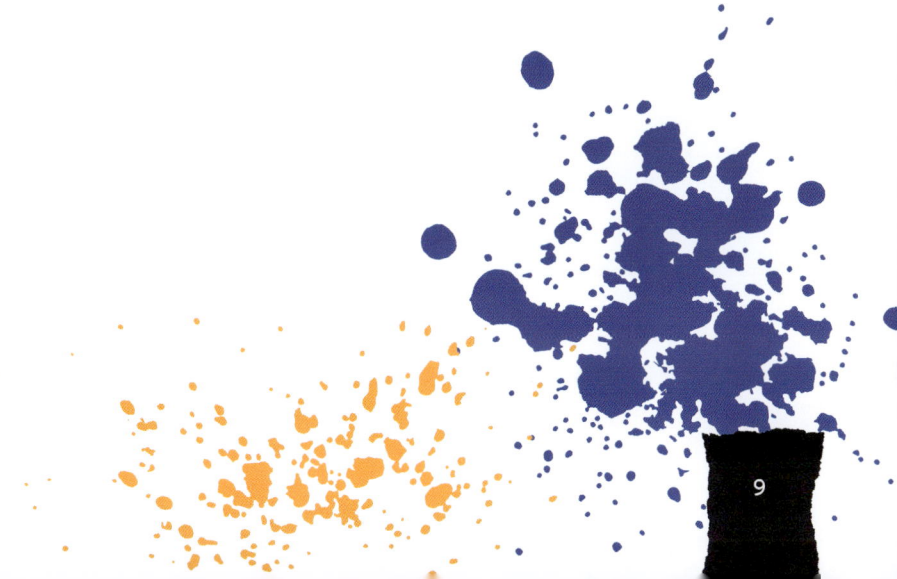

"Everyone should be able to get the support they need to bounce back from stroke."

— Dr. Shamala Thilarajah

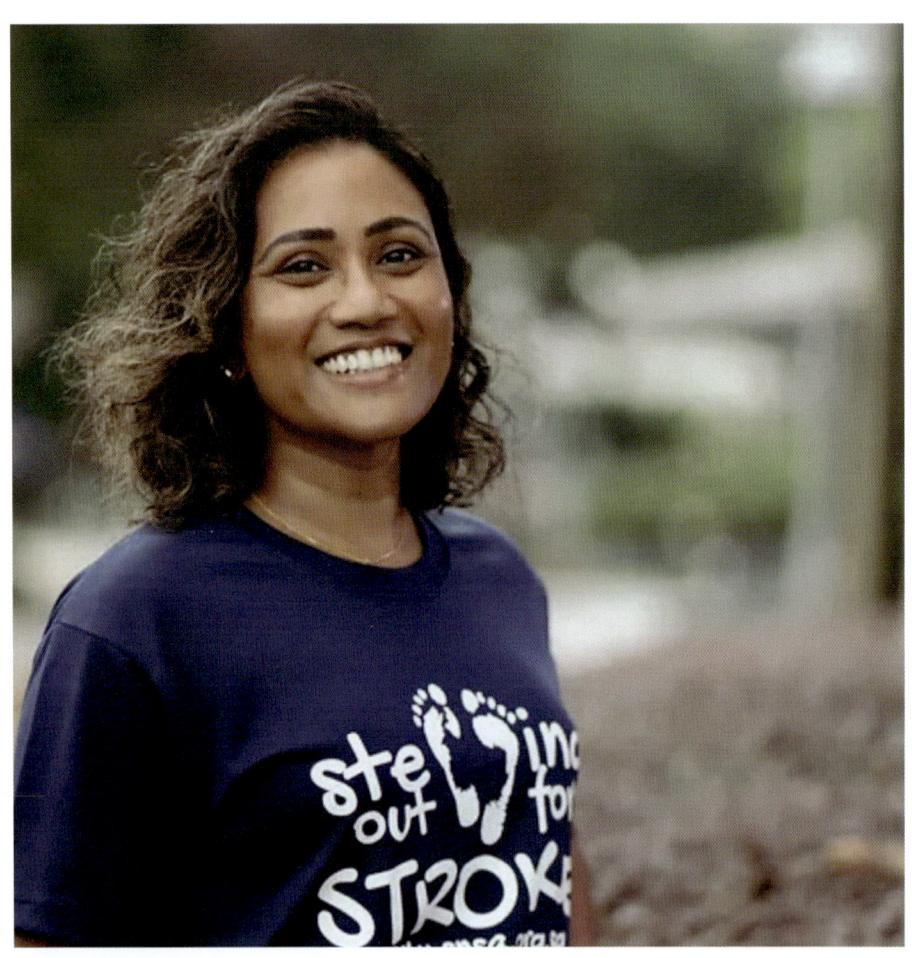

As both President of the Singapore National Stroke Association (SNSA) and a physiotherapist working in stroke rehabilitation, my work has provided me with an intimate understanding of the challenges stroke survivors encounter.

The prevalence of stroke, a leading global cause of disability, has been steadily increasing. In Singapore alone, the numbers have risen from 6,000 in 2010 to 8,000 today, profoundly impacting individuals, families, and communities. I have seen firsthand how formidable the condition can be; my own grandmother was also a stroke survivor, so this is something that especially hits home for me.

In my experience, particularly for outpatients in the recovery phase beyond six months, I have found that incorporating multicomponent exercises is crucial in keeping them healthy. The challenge lies in sticking to these exercise routines, which highlights the importance of accessible exercise options for stroke survivors, whether conducted at home, in facilities, or outdoors.

Collaborative efforts between healthcare professionals, government initiatives, and organisations such as SNSA are key to bridging the gap in accessibility to therapy. Community services such as the Stroke Support Station (S3), Abilities Beyond Limitations and Expectations (ABLE), and One-Rehab provide not only physical support but also avenues for mental wellness and social integration.

At SNSA, we advocate for a person-centric approach. This commitment to making a difference in the lives of those affected by stroke is upheld by our committed staff and volunteers. Thanks to government funding and grants, we have been able to touch the lives of over 3,000 (and counting) beneficiaries through our community involvement and stroke recovery programs in 2022.

Whether it is from family, friends, or peer support groups, having individuals who understand the journey can make all the difference. The importance of creating an environment where the individual feels encouraged and empowered to face each day cannot be overstated.

There is an urgent need for a sustainable model for long-term care and community integration for stroke survivors. With a comprehensive approach and ongoing support for survivors and their families, we can ensure that everyone affected will have the opportunity to bounce back and rebuild their lives after stroke.

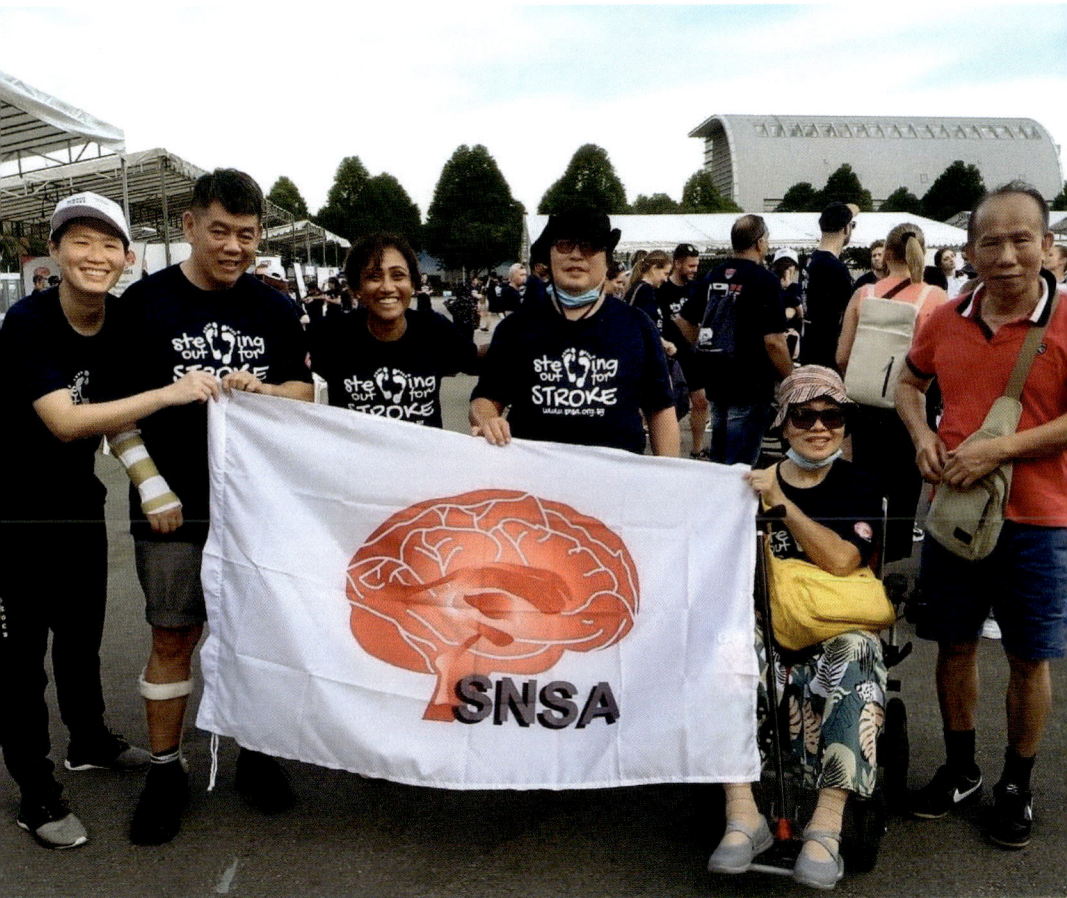

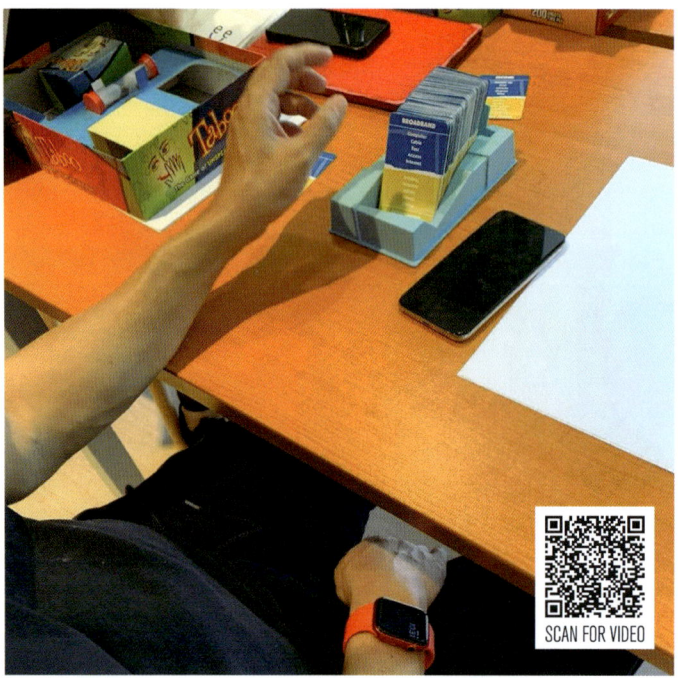

SCAN FOR VIDEO

Navigating the terrain of stroke rehabilitation unveils a realm of practice frequently overlooked: the nuanced exercise of speech. As I reflect on my journey thus far, I would be remiss not to highlight the impact speech therapy has had — a transformative process that played a significant role in helping me rediscover life on my own terms.

One of the most challenging aspects of
having aphasia, a result of stroke, is
the struggle to communicate. Imagine
a repository of thoughts and emotions
guarded by a key that stubbornly defies
functionality. Trying to speak often felt
like walking through thick fog, words
slipping away like shadows even though I was
trying my best.

Depression started to creep in when even
the people closest to me could not grasp the
extent of my difficulty with words. I went
into an emotional downward spiral, fuelled
by the frustration of my communication
difficulties.

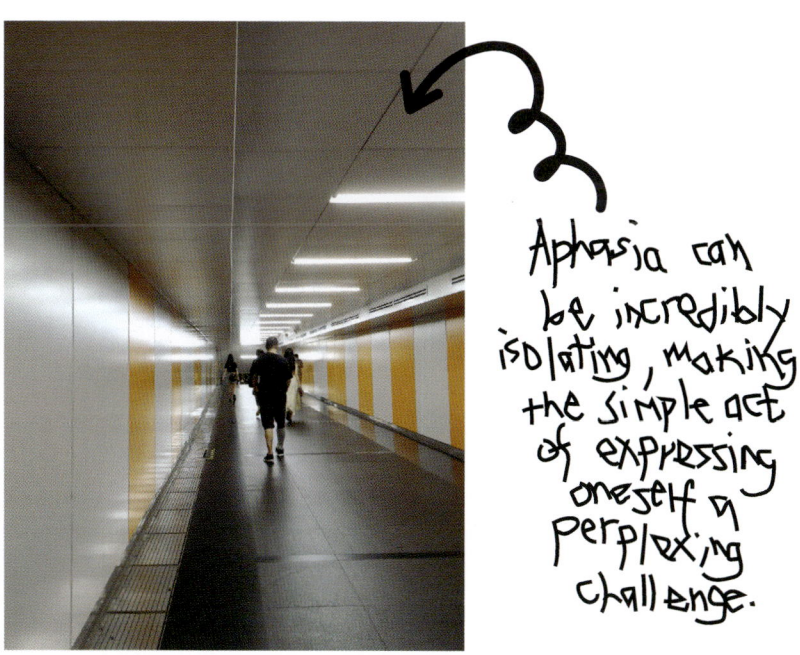

Aphasia can
be incredibly
isolating, making
the simple act
of expressing
oneself a
perplexing
challenge.

I would later learn that my experience was something backed by research. The heightened risk of depression amongst those grappling with aphasia is not just a coincidence but a consequence of losing connections with friends and support networks. When the bridge of language falters, the very relationships that used to offer comfort can turn into sources of despair.

Aphasia, with its disruptive impact on the neural pathways governing speech and language, necessitates a crucial intervention: speech therapy. I started working with speech and language therapist, Evelyn, who also founded Aphasia SG.

"Let's start with simple sounds," Evelyn would say, her voice tinged with encouragement. I then repeated things she said to me, each syllable a deliberate and conscious effort to reconnect my thoughts and the world outside. It was like a reprogramming of the brain, to navigate the maze of words once more.

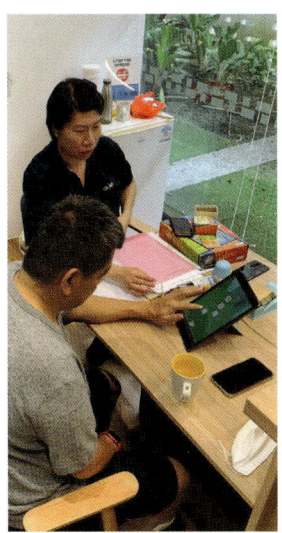

Much like the camaraderie found in a gym, the relationship between Evelyn and myself worked in similar fashion. She was not just an instructor but also a partner who was there for me, spurring and pushing me on to overcome my limitations.

Our sessions were filled with all kinds of exercises, from simple words to more complex sentence formations. The muscles involved in speech — my tongue, lips and vocal cords — all needed to be retrained. Each session felt akin to a trip to the linguistic gym, challenging me to lift the gruelling weight of aphasia.

Evelyn introduced me to different techniques to improve my communication skills. From word association games to picture cards, the activities were aimed towards helping me reclaim the language that had once flowed effortlessly from my lips.

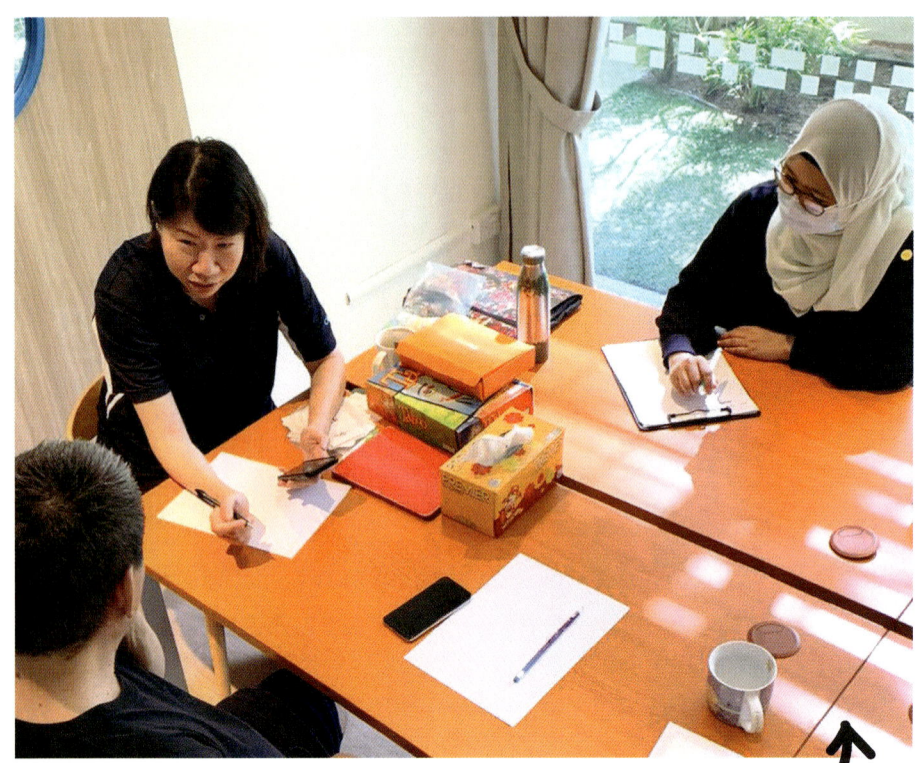

With Evelyn's help, the path to fluency was paved with unexpected moments of fun and laughter.

Initially, progress was slow, and frustration was an ever present spectre. Yet Evelyn's kindness and cheerful personality never let up. Whenever I struggled to articulate details, she patiently listened, offering words when my own failed me. She saw beyond the broken sentences and embraced the person beneath, an individual with a unique voice wanting to be heard.

Her office became a place where frustration melted away, and hope took its place. It was a safe space where I could stumble through the awkwardness of mispronunciations and incomplete sentences without fear of judgement. She had a knack especially for catering to my unique quirks, as well as infusing a sense of light-heartedness that made the sessions enjoyable.

Whether it was attending gatherings or participating in new activities, Evelyn's companionship provided a supportive backdrop. She invited me to join her at different events, gently coaxing me out of my comfort zone. I even managed to catch renowned author and playwright Lim Hai Yen at the launch of her beautiful book, *For Better, For Worse*.

Her story about stroke, too, deeply moved and resonated with me. Her eloquence and way with words was truly an inspiration — from one stroke survivor to another. I was extremely touched that she also took the time to write me this beautiful note after the event:

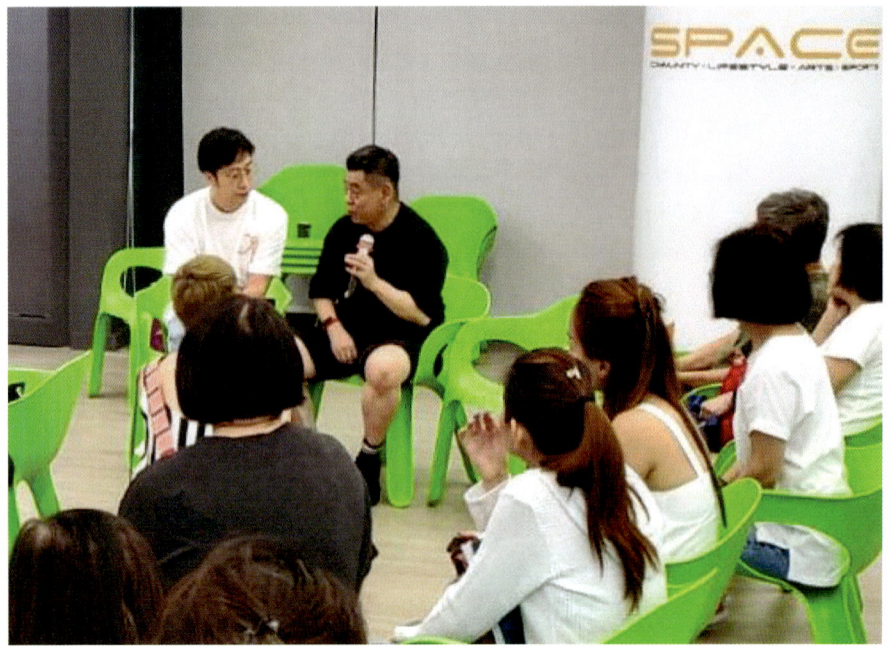

Terence is amazing!

He's a warrior — not willing to succumb to stark reality and fights back with gusto.

He's a survivor — not only wrote two books on his recovery of stroke but continues to deliver his third instalment.

He's a role model — his writing is frank and provides insights on overcoming adversity.

He is sincere, encouraging and down-to-earth. His books reflect his personality and demonstrate creativity not only in his writing and layout, but also in solving problems in life. I salute him for his passion and perseverance, in his pursuit of becoming a better and stronger person.

Terence turns setbacks into success!

Lim Hai Yen
Artistic Director, The ETCeteras,
Author, Playwright, Director, Drama Educator

Looking back, it was about embracing who I am and my own voice. I was reminded of the power language holds and the privilege and responsibility I had in penning my own books. No longer trying to fit in or sound like someone else, I was speaking for myself, and that was all that mattered. I had found a new rhythm and cadence that I cherished, one that was unique to me and my experiences.

The lessons learned in Evelyn's office echoed in my interactions with the world.

"Where the mind leads, the body follows."

— Evelyn Khoo

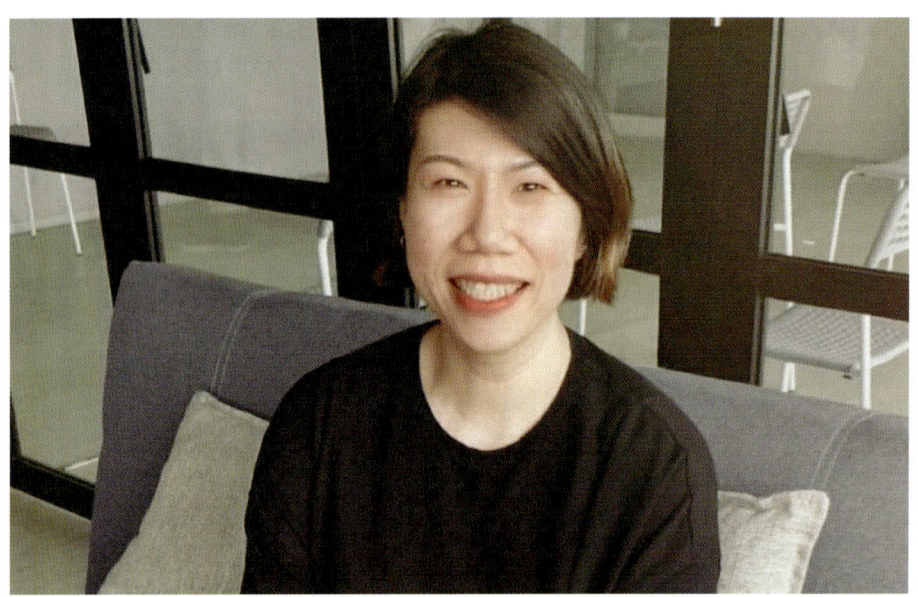

My role as a speech and language therapist allows me to work closely with people from all walks of life. The individuals I meet have diverse challenges, ranging from the complexities of aphasia to motor speech disorders to swallowing difficulties.

I often get asked "how do speech therapists treat patients with speech problems"? My response: "There is no magic pill or a one-size-fits-all programme."

Speech therapy involves a comprehensive assessment of the individual's speech, language, and swallowing abilities. With stroke patients, this includes evaluating the impact of neurological damage to the person's various functions. For example, if the stroke survivor suffered from motor speech impairment, we might teach them some physical exercises to strengthen their lips, tongue, and jaw muscles.

However, some patients with aphasia require other strategic approaches, such as training of communication partners to support their conversations. Therapy is, therefore, a personalised and collaborative process where we strive to understand patients' needs and goals, as well as identify their strengths and weaknesses, so that appropriate recommendations can be made.

I believe that a therapist should always consider the person's aspirations and implement interventions that allow them to regain confidence and reintegrate into society. This ensures that treatment is not only effective but also resonates meaningfully with the person's personal targets, increasing their motivation to keep working hard.

For instance, Terence, who thrives on visual stimuli, benefitted greatly from exercises capitalising on his strength of using visual association to improve working memory. When I first started working with Terence, he was very self-conscious about his speech and would sometimes stop talking out of frustration. Eventually, through a variety of language games and interactive activities like closed-door small group presentations, Terence was motivated to keep going and regained his confidence to speak in public.

Beyond my professional work, I am also passionate about volunteering and advocacy. Through Aphasia SG, I am connected with the wider community, and being a part of the aphasia support landscape in Singapore holds a special place in my heart.

Collaborating with volunteers has added a rich layer to this journey, and together, we have rolled out regular community initiatives for patients with aphasia and their caregivers. Our volunteers have also been tirelessly doing outreach activities to raise public awareness of aphasia.

Witnessing the growth of Aphasia SG brings me much joy to see a community where individuals dealing with aphasia can discover understanding and feel like they belong. It is my hope that through our collective advocacy, Singapore will become a truly inclusive society where persons with aphasia are treated with kindness and given the support they need in order to thrive.

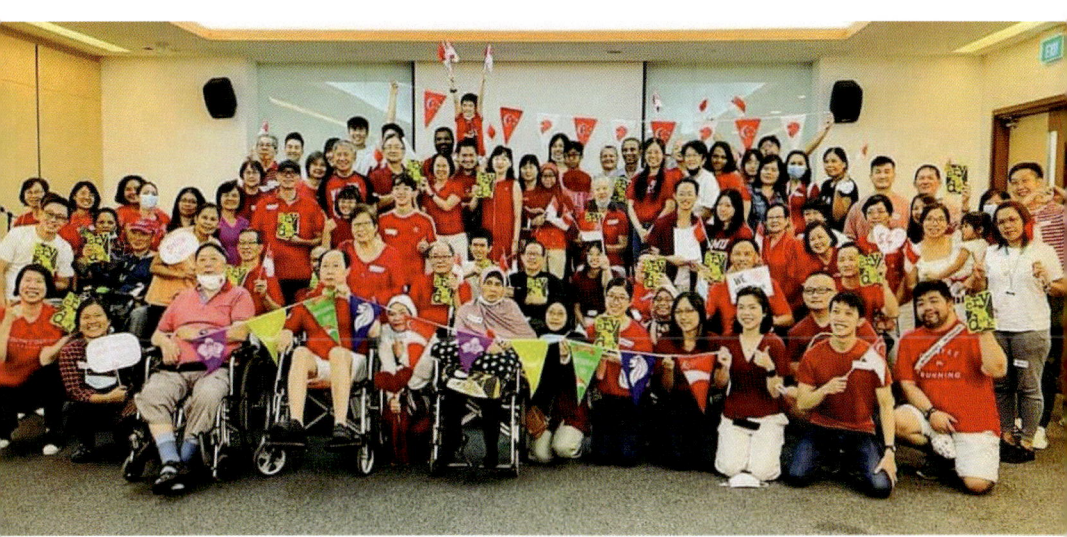

WORLD STROKE DAY 2022

My biggest adversary was always lurking within myself. It was not easy for me to admit that I needed help and initially, I waved off the helping hands extended by those genuinely concerned about my well-being. It took the steadfast support of many to pull me out from the gloom that self-pity had draped over my life.

Little did I expect it would lead me to a stage I never thought I would step onto — the World Stroke Congress. The idea of public speaking was, for me, a daunting prospect. I had always shied away from the spotlight, and the thought of speaking at a global event — what more a gathering of experts and healthcare professionals from all over the world — was something I had never considered.

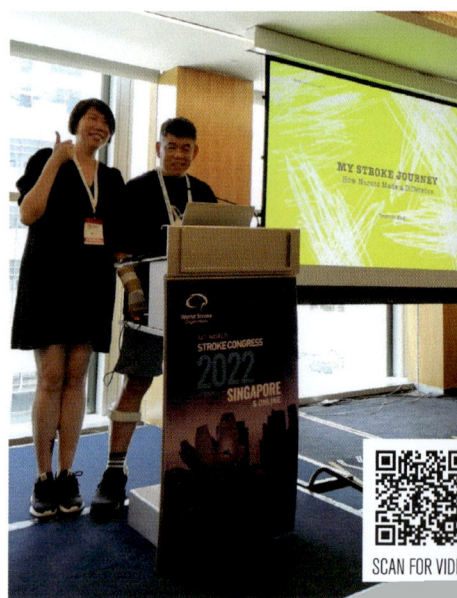

I was giving a speech on nurses and how they cared for me during my time in the hospital.

But sometimes, life takes unexpected turns, and this was one of those moments. Stepping into the hall and seeing the audience for the first time, I had second thoughts. I was unsure and nervous as I prepared, and had to remind myself of the support of my loved ones. I was not just speaking for myself — I was a representative of the stroke survivor community.

It was both humbling and empowering. And the response from the audience exceeded my expectations. Leading healthcare professionals approached me during breaks, expressing their appreciation for shedding light on the human side of stroke. Some shared personal stories of patients they had treated; their dedication to advancing medical science and improving patient care was palpable.

As I exchanged words with neurologists, therapists and researchers, I felt an uncanny sense of camaraderie. Despite our different roles in the healthcare ecosystem, we shared a common goal — the well-being of those affected by strokes.

The chance to contribute to the dialogue on stroke recovery was nothing short of awe-inspiring.

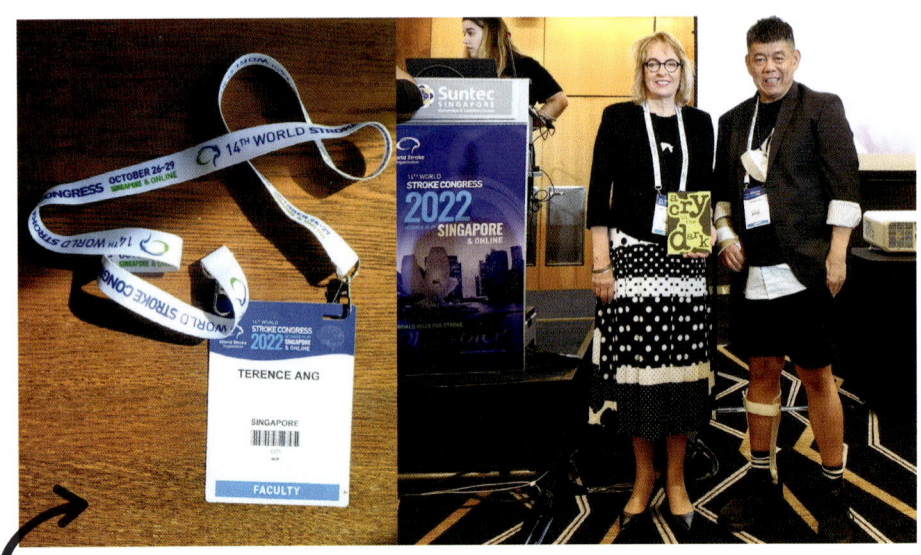

Meeting Professor Sandy Middleton, Director of the Nursing Research Institute at Australian Catholic University (ACU)!

What I had initially perceived as a personal journey through stroke was slowly evolving into a mission to help fellow stroke survivors. It was a moment of pride that extended beyond just overcoming the fear of public speaking. The World Stroke Congress showed me the power each of our voices holds, and its ability to inspire and effect changes.

As I continue on my journey of recovery, I am thankful for the people who supported me and helped me regain my voice. I may have lost a part of myself, but at the same time gained a newfound purpose — to use my experience to make a positive impact in the stroke community.

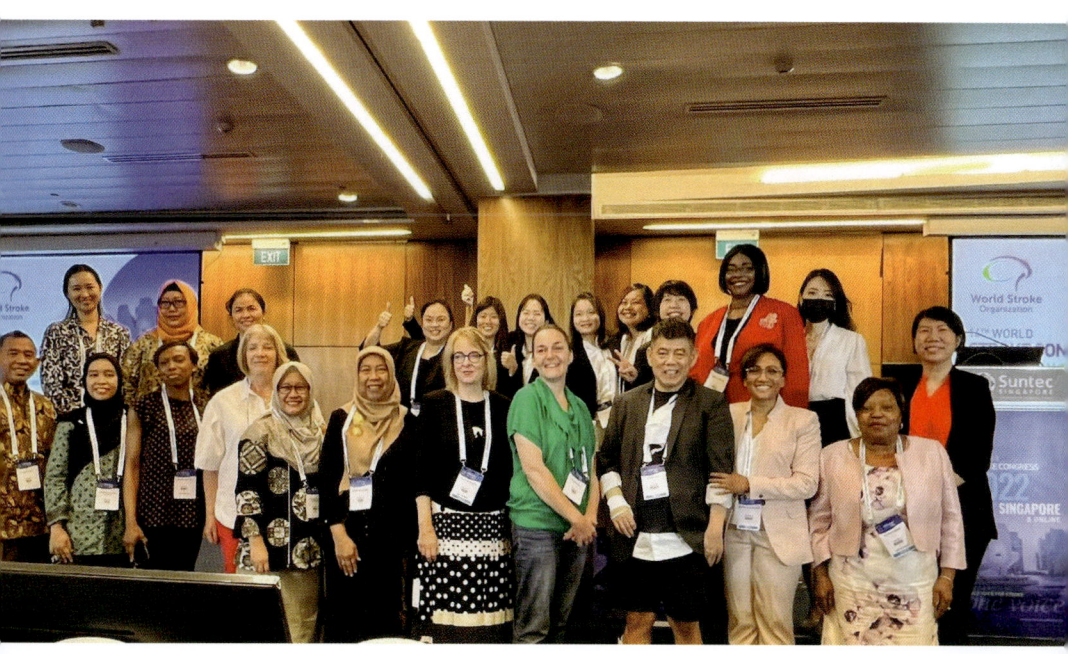

THE OCCUPATIONAL THERAPIST WHO CAN'T COUNT

My life before stroke was the epitome of the modern lifestyle. Exercise was never something I participated in, and the idea of breaking a sweat was simply not on my radar. I was content to stay within my comfort zone, blissfully ignorant to the consequences of a sedentary routine.

Work demanded long hours at the office glued to my desk, staring at a screen. Commuting to and fro was by car or public transportation. Evenings were spent in the cocoon of my living room and couch, where the television provided my primary source of entertainment.

Healthy eating was another foreign concept. I justified my poor dietary habits with excuses — I was too busy to cook, I deserved to treat myself after a long day, etc. It was not until much later that the significance of physical activity and its impact on our health really dawned on me.

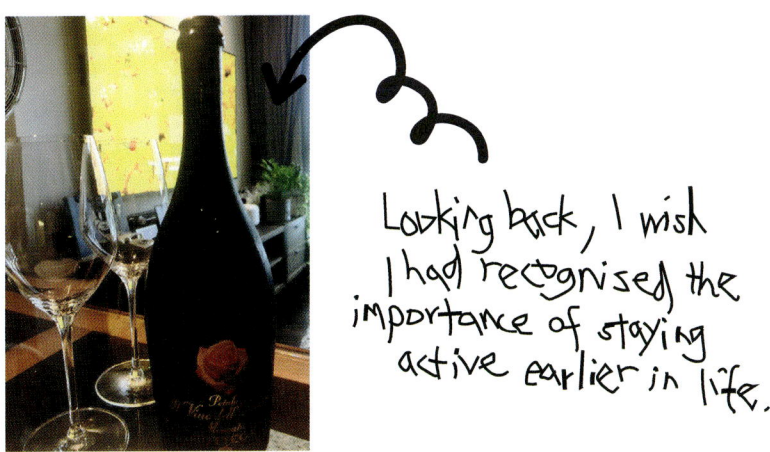

Looking back, I wish I had recognised the importance of staying active earlier in life.

The stroke was a jarring wake-up call, a reminder that everything can change in an instant. Simple tasks that I once took for granted became formidable challenges. Most days, I felt powerless and disheartened. I had to think a lot about each step I took. My independence had evaporated.

Wednesdays and Saturdays became my designated days for occupational therapy, something I always looked forward to. In hindsight, it is remarkable how Sijie, my occupational therapist, has been a constant in my life for over a year now, helping me out of that dark period.

Occupational therapy, as it turns out, is not just exercises performed for the sake of physical activity. Rather, it focuses on practical skills, addressing the specific day-to-day challenges individuals face. We worked on a wide range of exercises aimed at enhancing my motor skills and restoring functionality to crucial areas such as my wrist and hand mobility.

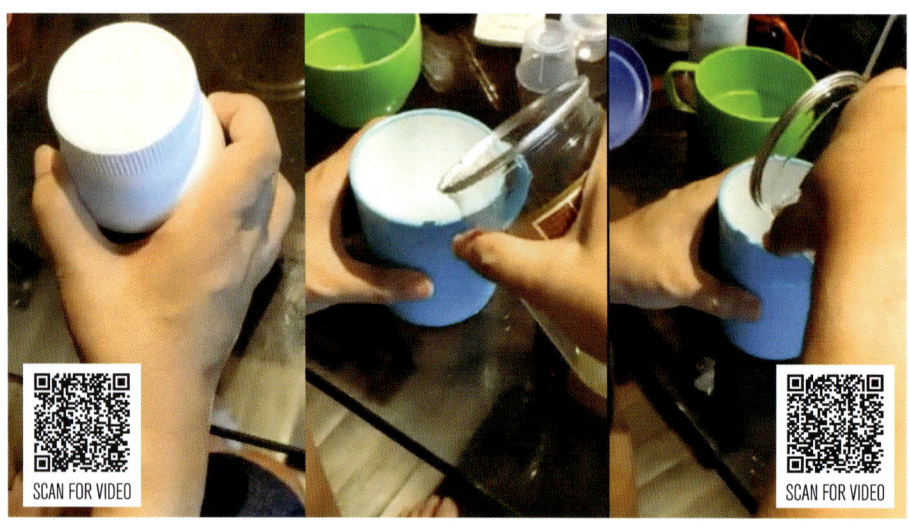

SCAN FOR VIDEO

SCAN FOR VIDEO

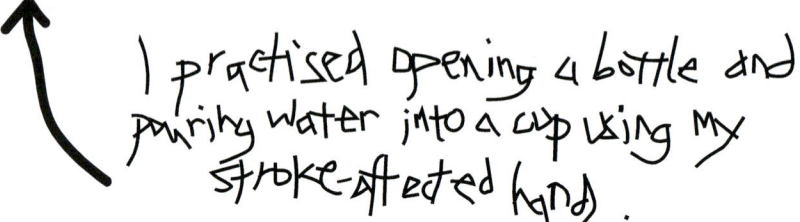

I practised opening a bottle and pouring water into a cup using my stroke-affected hand.

Could I straighten my arm? Could I coordinate my movements? These were things we tackled. Sijie helped me to set small goals for each session, and each time I reached one, he would encourage me to keep pushing forward. I always felt more capable and empowered each time I completed a task.

Over time, we developed a unique rapport. I discovered that Sijie is a bit of a character, often bringing a playful energy to our sessions that I greatly appreciate. Occasionally, he will joke about not coming anymore and leaving me to fend for myself, but I can see the twinkle in his eyes, and I know he genuinely cares. It is his way of keeping the atmosphere casual and stress-free, and we will always have a good laugh.

Tension gliding exercises as well as pronation stretches were targeted towards the rotational movements of my forearms.

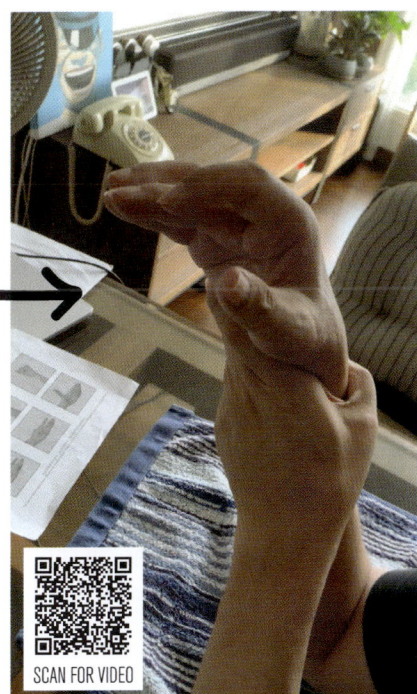

I think what made the process even more special was that Sijie and I just naturally understood each other. He was not merely guiding me through exercises; he was also great at making therapy meaningful, relevant and uplifting.

"Excuse me, hello, both hands," he would say as he caught me slipping back into the familiarity of relying on my good hand. The key was to get me using my stroke-affected hand more, whether it was picking stuff up, using my phone, or anything under the sun.

For one, typing was something I faced much difficulty with every day. We worked on typing exercises, and while it may seem like a simple task to most, it was endlessly frustrating for me. Every time I rested, my fingers would slide and tremble. It was most inconvenient and discouraging.

Sijie then introduced me to Oval 8 splints that immobilised my fingers and made the exercise more manageable. He always comes up with these interesting ideas, turning our sessions into new and exciting adventures. I cannot help marvelling at his resourcefulness, but here is something funny about him on that note — his seeming inability to count.

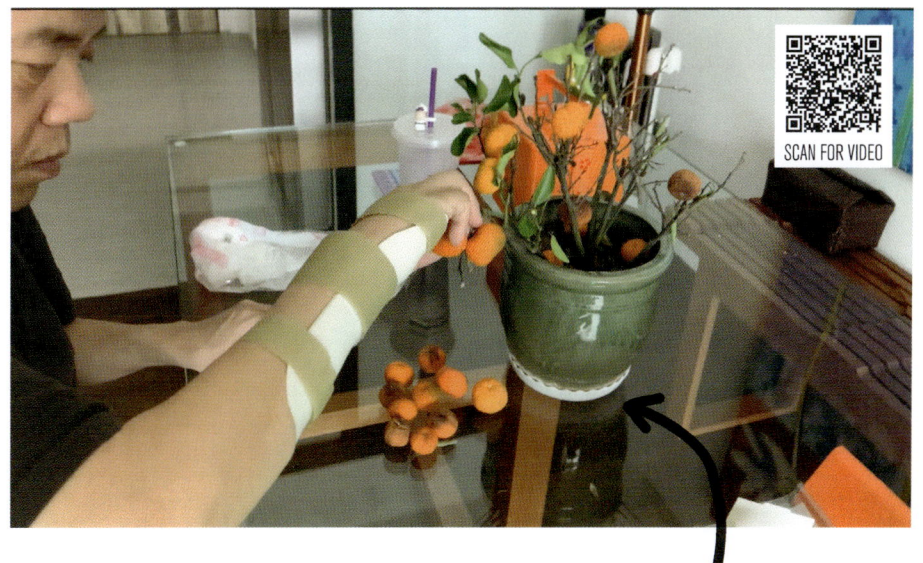

SCAN FOR VIDEO

Sijie often makes use of the everyday stuff in my home, here, he has me doing fine motor training through picking oranges.

I have been noticing for a while that Sijie would frequently lose track of how many repetitions we have done for an activity, and it forced me to be extra vigilant, trying to keep count in my head. As I grunted through a particularly strenuous task, Sijie's number counting would become increasingly erratic, "Three… four… two… uh, what was it again, just do five more!" I groaned, but did as I was told, even though I thought I was done.

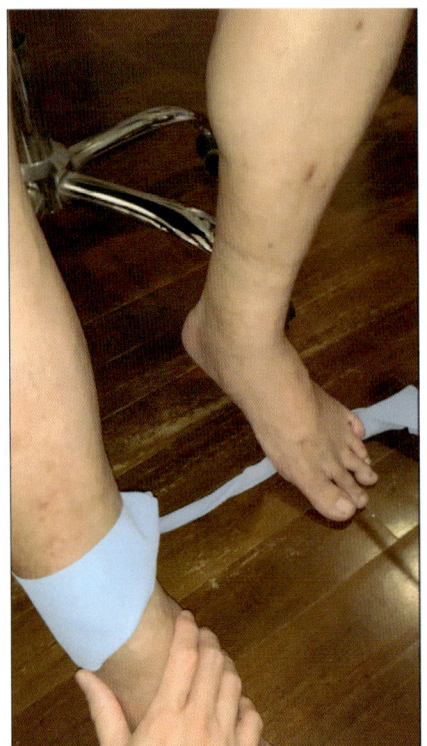 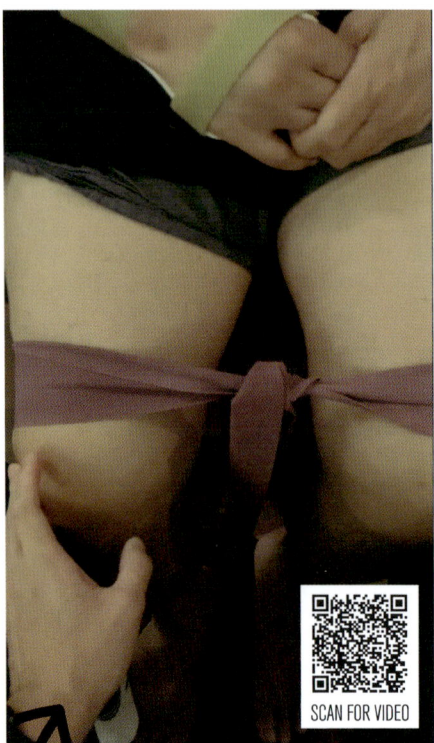

These hip flexion and adduction
exercises are more tiring than they
look!

Most of the time though, his "forgetfulness" when counting appeared to be a deliberate strategy, as if he had a secret plan to get me to do more of everything. I learned to adapt to Sijie's unpredictable counts, in part because I knew he only meant the best for me. It became a unique part of our dynamic, one of our many shared inside jokes.

I think the thing I like most about Sijie is that he does not sugarcoat things or beat around the bush. He tells it like it is. And while some may not appreciate it, it is exactly what I need. I never felt like he was giving up on me or telling me something just to get me to feel better. Instead, he challenges me every step of the way.

There were times when I felt stuck, but Sijie reminded me that it was okay to take it one day at a time. When I am feeling particularly down or disheartened, he would take the time to sit with me and talk. He never tries to downplay my feelings and is always willing to adjust our sessions based on areas where I need improvement.

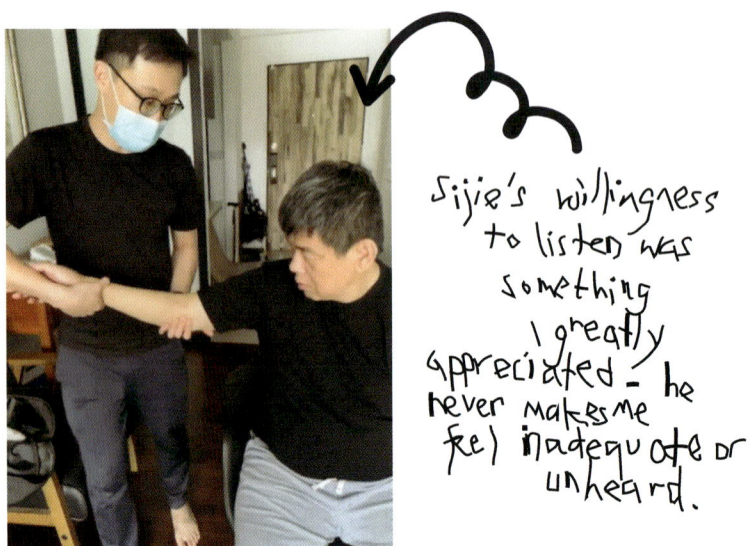

Sijie's willingness to listen was something I greatly appreciated - he never makes me feel inadequate or unheard.

It is in moments like these that make the sessions feel more of a reunion with an old friend rather than a therapy appointment. Sijie, the "bitch" (as I affectionately call him), has undoubtedly played a vital role in guiding me through my stroke story.

STROKE AND AFTERCARE

When it comes to post-stroke rehabilitation, there are many scenarios where patients find themselves at a crossroads, no longer receiving therapy. This can be due to several factors, and it raises important questions about what comes next in their journey.

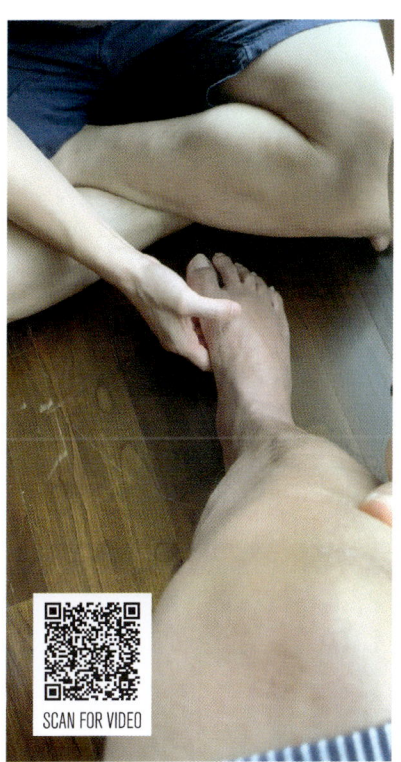

SCAN FOR VIDEO

One common scenario is when patients are discharged from the hospital without receiving further therapy. In restructured hospitals, the main focus is on treating and discharging patients home timely. There is not always enough time for deep conversations about long-term recovery.

The length of stay in a neurological ward, typically 1-3 weeks depending on severity, or 4-6 weeks in inpatient rehabilitation programs, can be relatively short in the grand scheme of things. Therapists often meet their short-term goals within these time frames, but patients may not have fully achieved their potential recovery.

Although the assumption may be that they have reached a point where they can continue their recovery independently, the reality is that having a stroke is often a chronic condition. Many patients still have areas they need to work on, even after their hospital stay.

Some may find themselves receiving therapy at outpatient clinics or day rehab centres. While certain individuals do make progress, most continue to face challenges. There are also cases where patients do not feel empowered to share about what is going on, asserting that they are "okay already", even if there is more to be done. They may not even realise they have a voice in their treatment decisions.

It is a problem that is multifold, but the main thing to remember is that you have to take charge of your own life and health. It is easy to become complacent and too dependent on your therapists and healthcare providers. You have to be your own advocate.

To that end, this ownership thing is not just on the patient — it is a team effort, and family plays a big role. Therapists, armed with a comprehensive understanding of the patient's life and context, are equally indispensable in delivering the best aftercare. It also falls on the community and our healthcare providers to bridge this gap.

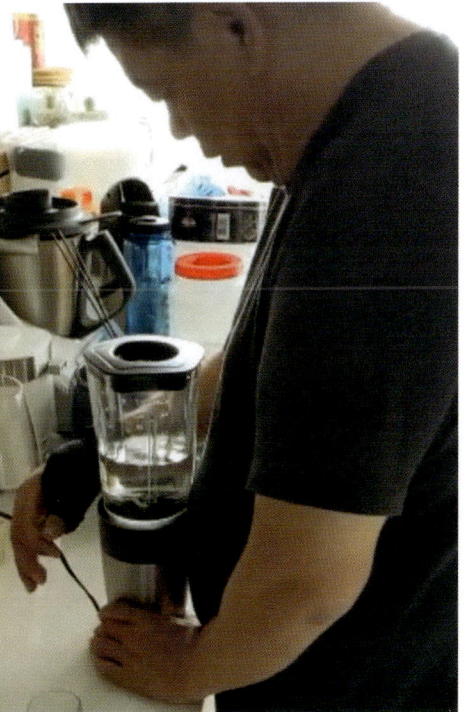

One of the things I found particularly helpful was practising how to use a blender again — healthy shakes, here I come!

We must recognise the ongoing and
evolving nature of stroke recovery
and find appropriate times to discuss
patients' needs and goals. By fostering
a collaborative and informed approach,
we pave the way for an environment where
recovery becomes not just a possibility but
a shared endeavour that encompasses the
entire spectrum of the patient's life.

"How many was that? Never mind,
do 5 more reps again."

— Sijie Lin

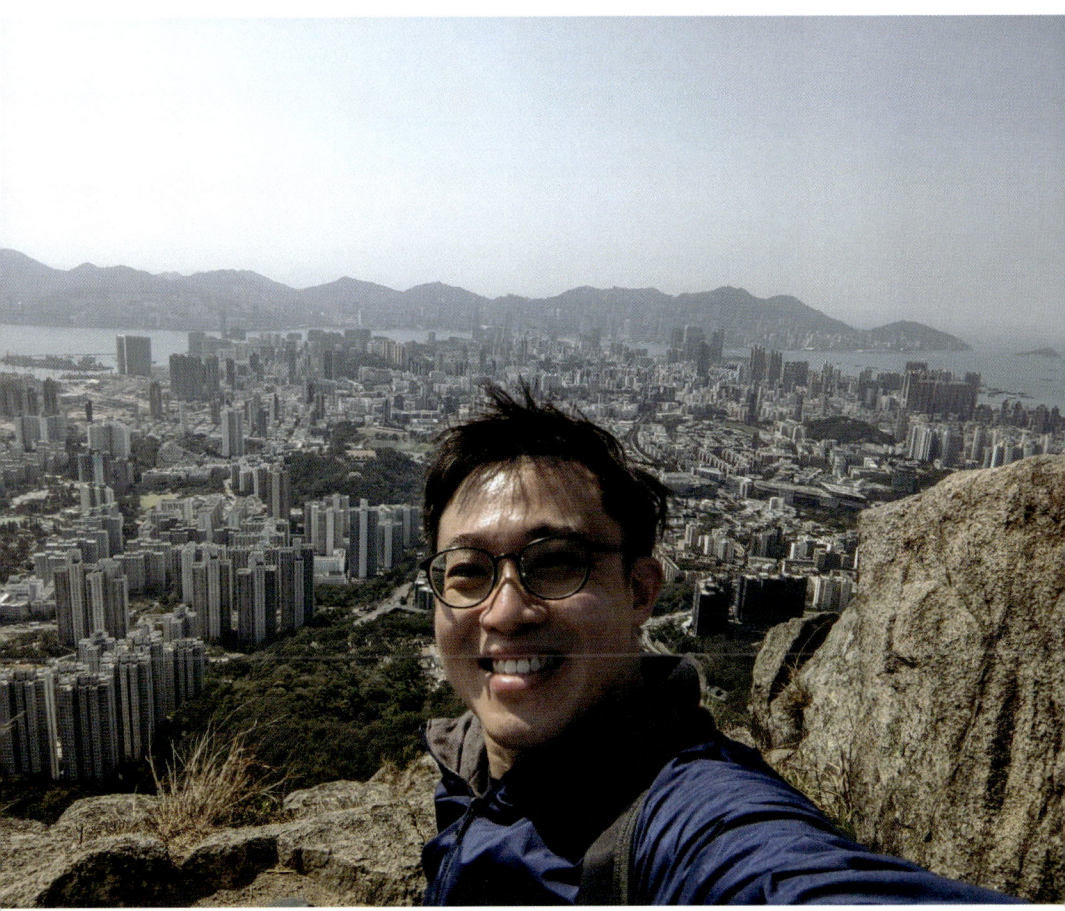

My journey into occupational therapy (OT) was not straightforward. Although it initially began as a backup plan, it later turned into a source of genuine joy and purpose. I pursued a diploma in occupational therapy at Nanyang Polytechnic (NYP) School of Health Sciences, where I learned about the profound impact OT can have on stroke rehab.

I see OT as distinct from physiotherapy (PT). We focus more on facilitating life skills to promote independence, understanding what is important to the patient, which, in turn, helps them regain participation in what they enjoy. Some of the many key aspects of my therapy involves identifying issues or barriers — be it physical, psychosocial or environmental — and modifying activities to boost participation in therapy sessions, as well as learning what is important to the patient and the goals they want to achieve through the rehab journey.

The journey through rehab is often a long one, and it can be challenging as patients struggle with their recovery. Effective communication and sustaining motivation become pivotal, especially when confronted with setbacks and the weight of personal expectations. Each day brings its own set of challenges, and it is on those harder days that the true strength of my patients is tested.

One of these instances was when Terence suffered his fall a year ago. We were both naturally disappointed as we were only just starting to make progress together. The fall not only hindered his physical mobility but also dealt a blow to his confidence, making the journey ahead seem even more daunting.

I remember the first walk I convinced Terence to take after the accident. It might seem like a small thing, but it felt like a huge win. Despite the challenges, Terence showed amazing determination to get stronger and move better.

What stood out even more was Terence's sense of humour. Even when things were tough, he stayed positive, which can make a big difference. With each session, I noticed small changes beginning to take place. It is a great example that reminds me how rehab can bring back strength and hope and a fresh start.

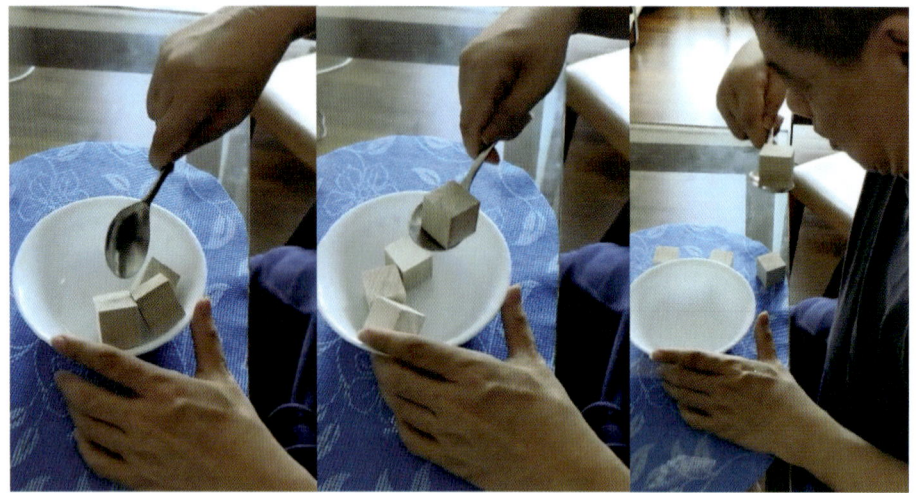

Throughout my journey as an occupational therapist, I have realised that it is a role that demands not only medical expertise but also empathy, patience, and a genuine desire to help individuals regain control over their lives. The rehab phase is important, but so is aftercare, knowing about the existing support systems, and how patients can continue their progress beyond our sessions.

We want to make sure people have the tools and support they need to keep moving forward. By spreading awareness and putting effective programs in place, we are helping stroke survivors to lead happy and independent lives outside of therapy.

TOUGH LOVE

I do not just want to be the best; I need
it. The standards I set for myself are
relentless and unforgiving. It is not
enough for me to succeed; I must excel.

As far as I can remember, pursuing
perfection has always been my driving
force. Whatever I set my mind to, I give
my 200 per cent. Anything less than that
is a failure, a bitter disappointment that
leaves a sour taste in my mouth.

This has, for better or worse, seeped
into every facet of my life. Whether it is
in my career, personal relationships or
endeavours, I cannot help but strive for
excellence. I want the best — I must be the
best.

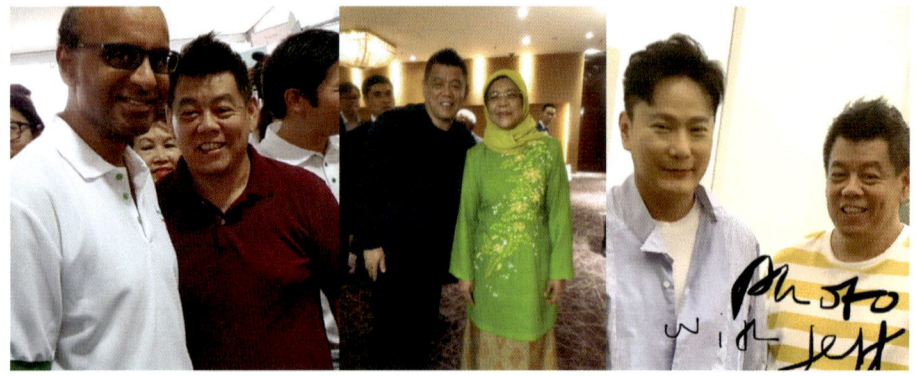

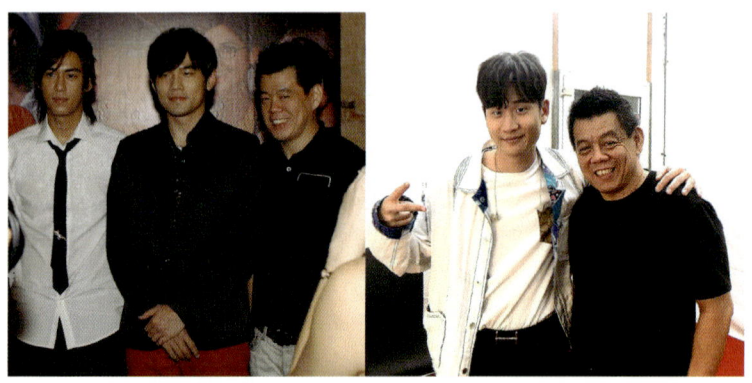

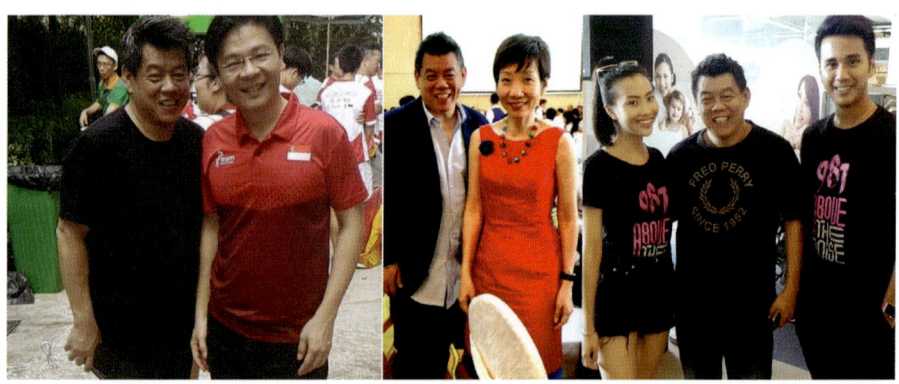

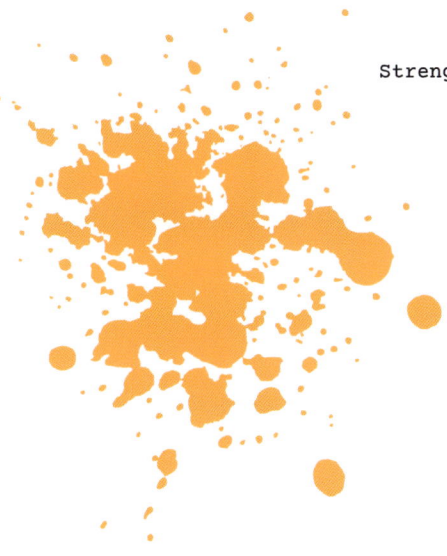

Living life in the fastlane — spot the famous faces I met along the way . . .

Mr Tharman Shanmugaratnam – President of Singapore,

Mdm Halimah Yacob – Former President of Singapore,

Jeff Chang – Taiwanese Singer and Actor

Baron Chen – Taiwanese Actor and Model,

Jay Chou – Taiwanese Singer and Musician,

Eric Chou – Taiwanese Singer and Actor

Mr Lawrence Wong – Deputy Prime Minister of Singapore,

Ms Grace Fu – Minister for Sustainability and the Environment of Singapore,

Sonia Chew and Joakim Gomez – Singaporean Radio Presenters

One of the people I met on my journey was Kha Seng, a personal trainer referred to me by my physiotherapist, Steve. Kha Seng's presence was magnetic — he had that kind of physique and confidence that commanded both respect and envy. As a former bodybuilder and fitness enthusiast himself, his approach to personal training was anything but ordinary.

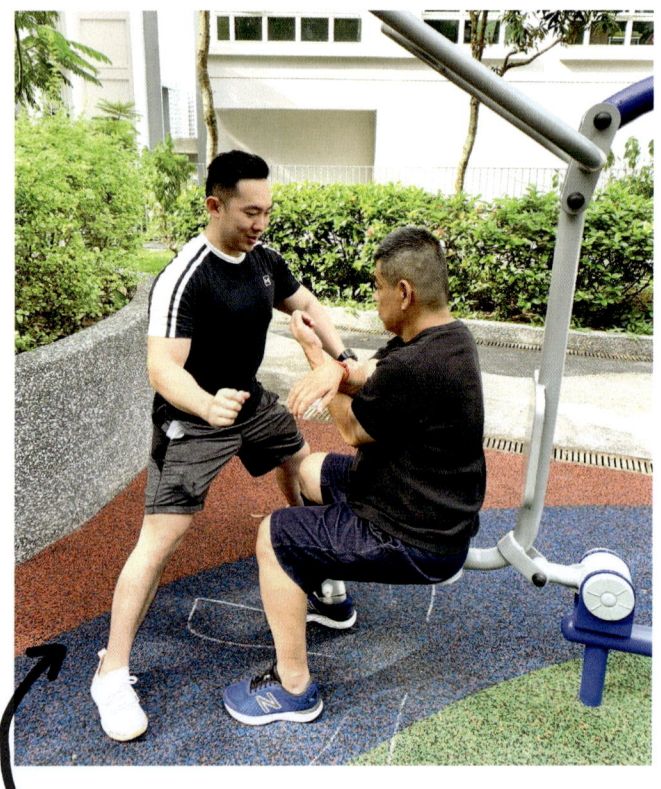

Your favourite work out playlist's energy packed in one muscle magician!

Kha Seng understood the unique challenges stroke survivors faced and that cookie-cutter solutions would not suffice. We discussed my goals in painstaking detail, and with that information, Kha Seng came up with a training plan.

Our sessions were twice a week, and he made sure I did not have an easy way out. Rain or shine, we would find a way to train. When it rained, he would suggest we take the stairs to the second floor of the sheltered car park, just to make sure I could not "siam" (evade the workout).

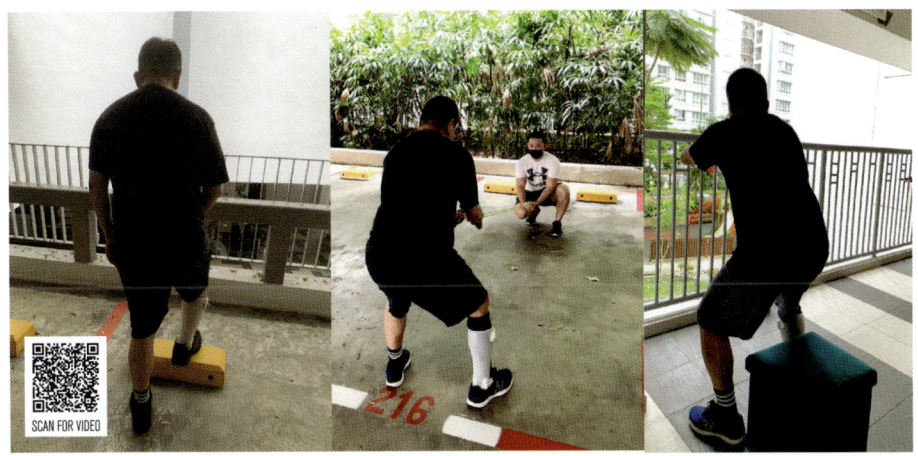

Doing squats and stepping up curbs outdoors; where I saw limitations, Kha Seng saw potential.

In the early days, every session was a test of my determination. There were moments when I wanted to give up. I questioned my sanity and commitment, and most of the time, I found myself struggling.

Some days, there was eagerness to challenge myself. On others, I was simply too tired or unmotivated to participate. But Kha Seng would not allow me to settle for less. He told me stories of people who had overcome incredible odds and achieved remarkable feats. I, too, believed I could be one of them.

For me, my focus was on building power in my legs. We started with basic exercises like stepping up and squatting with the aid of a portable chair for support. As my strength grew, we gradually removed the support. Kha Seng emphasised the crucial connection between the mind and muscles, instilling in me a heightened awareness of my body.

Although progress was slow, I could observe changes starting to happen. I had slowly grown stronger and fitter than people who did not exercise regularly. It spoke volumes to the effectiveness of Kah Seng's training plan and how, with the right guidance, individuals have the power to take charge of their lives.

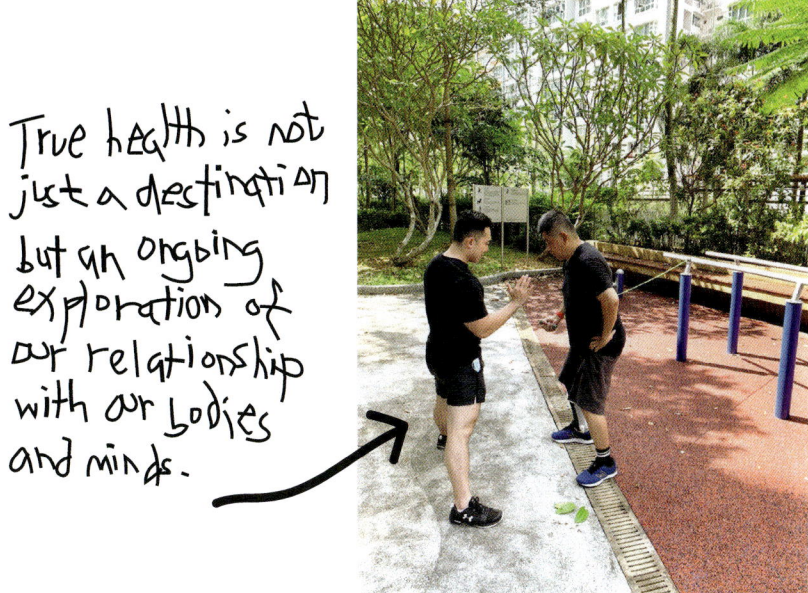

True health is not just a destination but an ongoing exploration of our relationship with our bodies and minds.

Two years ago, if someone had told me about the progress I would make, I would have found it hard to believe. Back then, I was uncertain about what the future held, struggling just to regain basic mobility. Now, I am more energetic, independent and confident.

It was Kah Seng's mission to improve lives, and it falls upon me to be grateful for the support and resources I have, knowing that there are others who are in worse situations than mine. As I let go of the unrealistic standards I had set for myself, I found that my journey became more meaningful in turn.

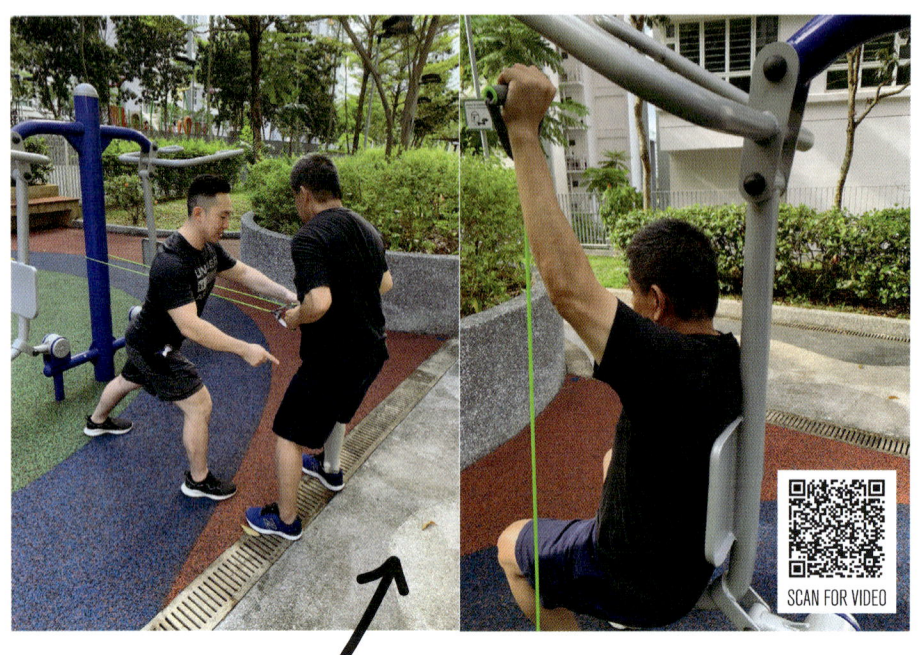

SCAN FOR VIDEO

My quality of life has improved, and I feel more vibrant and alive.

Allowing myself to make mistakes and learn from my missteps was a liberating feeling. It was as if a weight I had carried for years had been lifted from my shoulders. And it was a shift in perspective that enriched my life in many unexpected ways.

THE ART OF PERSONAL TRAINING

Stroke treatment often involves
working with a physical or
occupational therapist. While
the conventional approach
primarily focuses on restoring
physical function, personal
training can play a
transformative secondary
role. By providing support and
motivation beyond the physical
elements, what it does is offer
a fresh and holistic perspective.

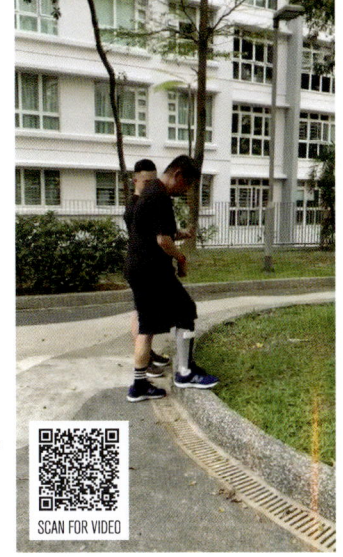

SCAN FOR VIDEO

A personal trainer serves not
just as an instructor but as a
motivator (and emotional boost)
too. They inspire and create safe spaces
for individuals to explore their potential,
physically and mentally. Confidence, once
shaken, finds solid ground in this empowering
relationship, reshaping perceptions of what
is achievable post-stroke.

Stroke survivors often face challenges that can limit their ability to attend regular gym sessions. Mobility issues, transportation constraints, or personal preferences are just a few that can hinder consistent access to fitness facilities. To that end, a home-based exercise program was something that worked for me.

Creating a home-based exercise program involves the consideration of equipment accessibility. The goal is to design routines that require minimal equipment or utilise things commonly found in the home or neighbourhood. This approach not only makes the exercises feasible but helps participants to integrate their workout routines into daily life.

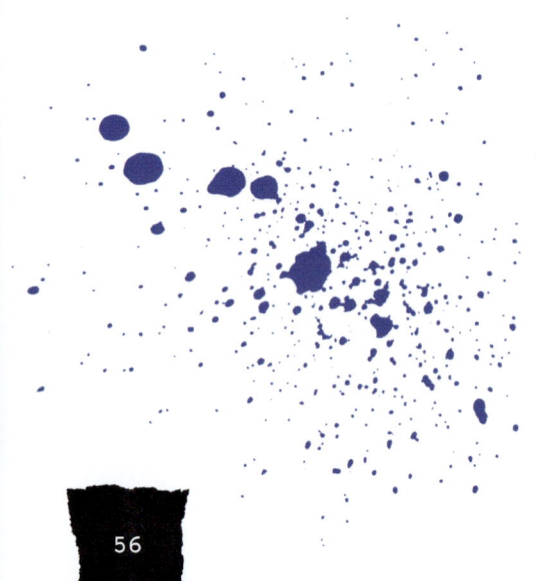

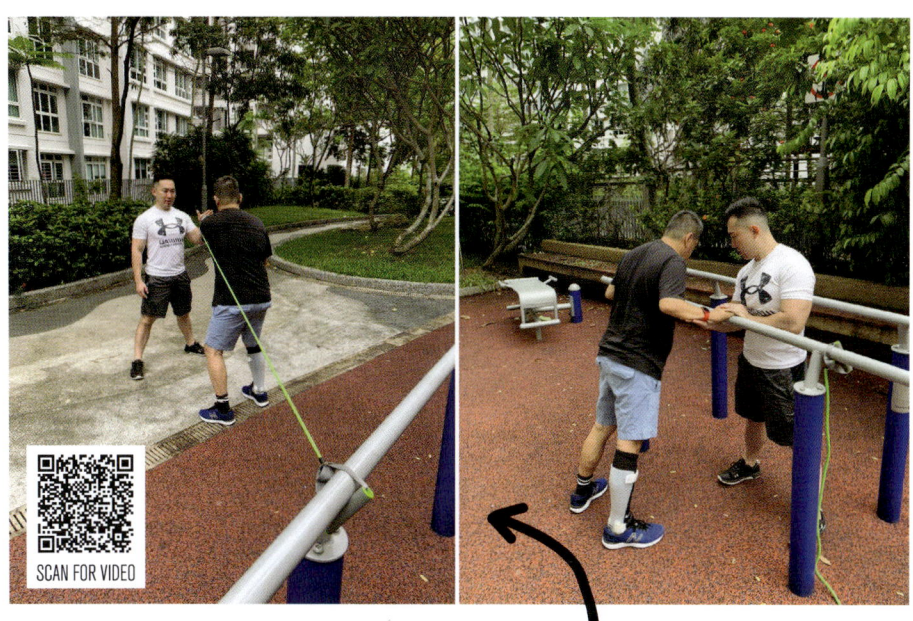

SCAN FOR VIDEO

Turning the park into a gym! Standing single arm chest file with resistance, chest push up on bars.

Regular check-ins with a personal trainer not only helps to track physical progress but also allows for exercise plans to adapt for evolving needs. This ongoing dialogue establishes a sense of accountability, and encourages active participation. As milestones are conquered, new goals can be set, shaping a continuous journey that resonates with the individual's changing needs and aspirations.

"Ready? Strike a pose and squeeze!"

— Tan Kha Seng

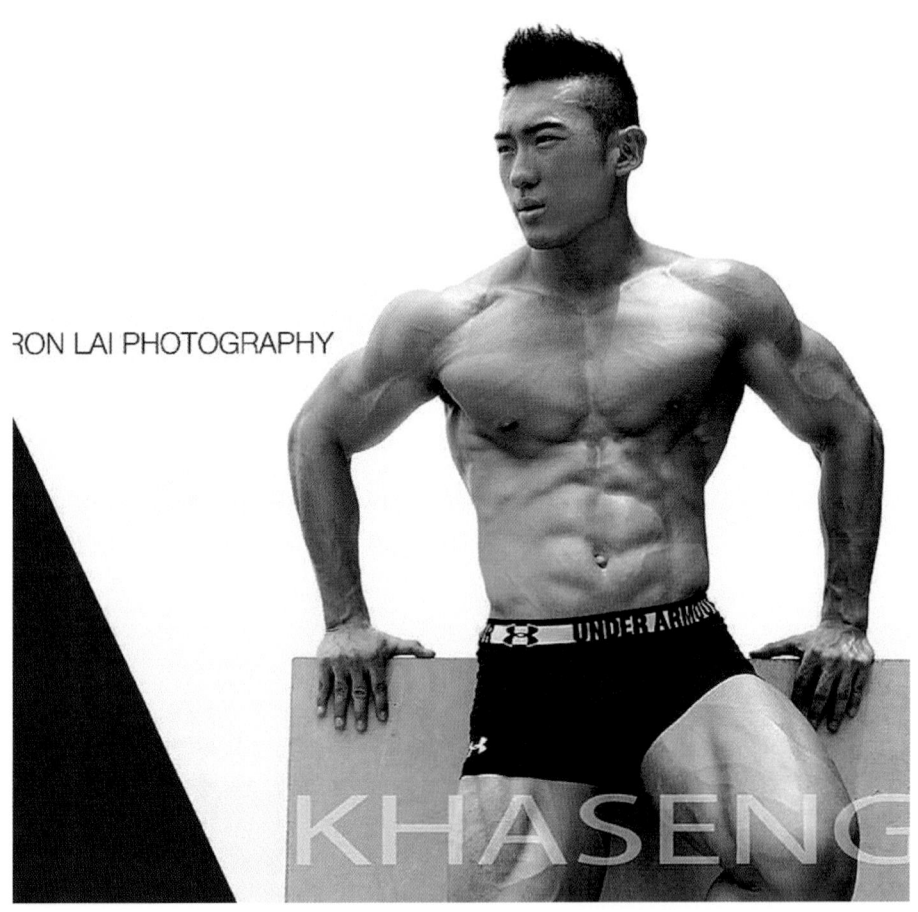

In my personal fitness journey, the goal has always been beyond the aesthetic appeal. Personal training is not only about achieving a certain look. It also helps to improve one's lifestyle and confidence. And regular sessions, even twice a week, can significantly enhance strength and overall fitness.

I find that motivating clients to actively participate in their fitness journey is pivotal in contributing to their success. Equally important is the management of expectations and setting attainable goals while accentuating the positive shifts. This instils a sense of accomplishment and fosters a commitment to enduring progress.

Yet it is also important to recognise that doing exercises improperly can lead to more harm than good. Each person's fitness capacity and body type define the path we take, and to me, the real deal is quality training that is safe and effective. Understanding individual needs is necessary in determining a suitable training regimen.

When working with stroke patients like Terence, safety is especially important, so there was a need to adjust the exercises accordingly. We focused a lot on building power in his legs through strength training, and also targeted exercises to improve his flexibility and mobility. I closely monitored his form and ensured that he maintained proper alignment and correct technique. It was crucial to prevent any unnecessary strain or risk of injury.

Throughout Terence's training, he has shown remarkable dedication and resilience. Slowly, we increased the range of motion over time to help him regain his mobility. Witnessing his progress, however gradual, has been incredibly rewarding. It was a privilege to play a part in his journey.

The satisfaction of aiding people in realising their fitness aspirations and witnessing their transformations is what drives me every day. It is a reminder of the value personal training holds, helping people build stronger bodies, prevent ailments, and ultimately lead better lives.

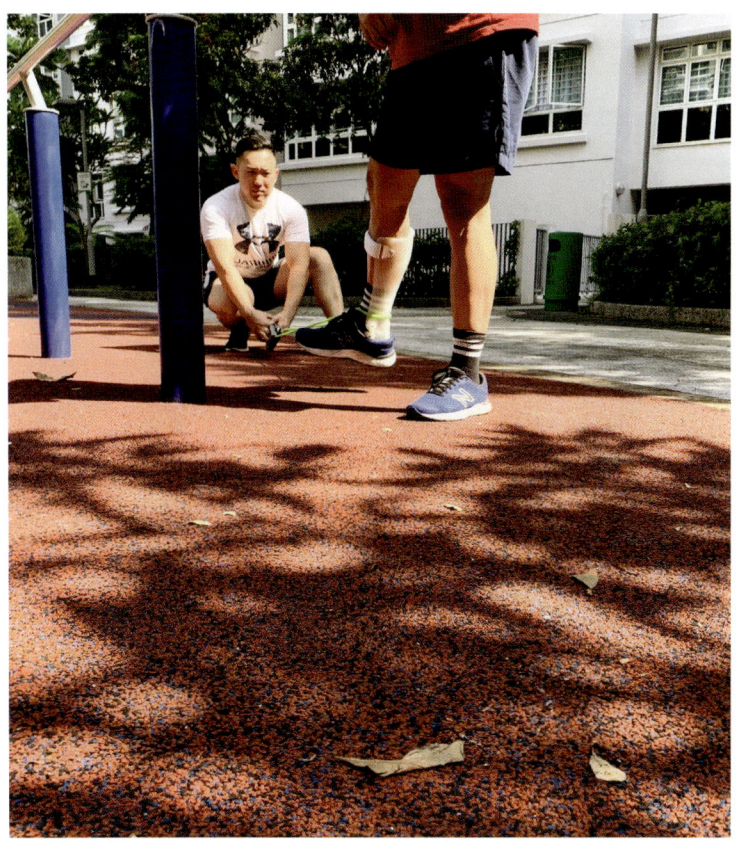

When clients look forward to the next
session with genuine enthusiasm, I know
I have hit the mark. It is creating a
positive association with exercise, making
it something they choose to embrace — not
because they have to, but because they
genuinely want to. That is when I know I am
making a real difference.

HELP! I'VE FALLEN AND CAN'T GET BACK UP

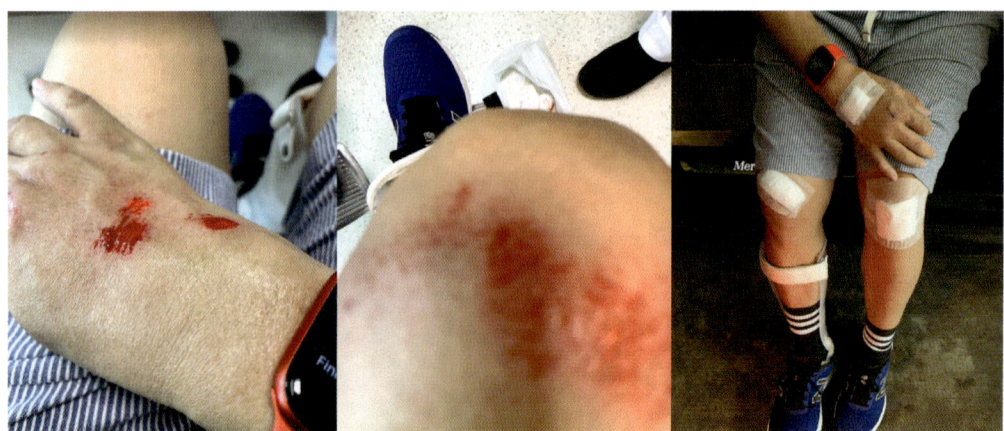

It was as if the ground had been pulled out from under my feet. Laying there sprawled on the unforgiving pavement, what seemed like an eternity must have passed. A fleeting moment, a slip, a loss of footing, and the world seemed to tilt on its axis.

I considered myself tough, having gone through the stroke with what I believed was a decent amount of grit. But the fall dispelled that notion, exposing the vulnerability beneath my strength.

My body, already weakened from the long battle, struggled to cope with this new blow. The pain was excruciating, but the emotional toll was even heavier. It had somehow found a way to leave me more debilitated than before.

So I chose the sanctuary of my home, retreating within its familiar walls and into an infinite hiatus from society. I wanted to shield myself from the prying and unkind gazes I thought awaited me; that was not something I had the capacity to deal with.

Days turned into weeks, and weeks into months, as the world outside moved on without me. I remained confined within the four walls that had witnessed the chronicles of my life. There was a lot of time to think, too much time to ponder. Would I ever regain the ability to walk without stumbling? Could I really keep doing this? Was I doomed to be stuck in the shadows of my limitations?

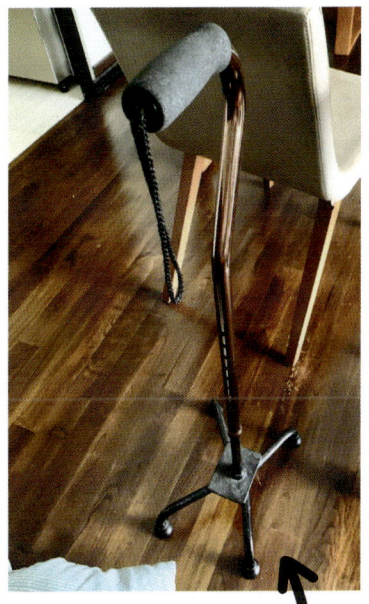

life got a bit tangled, doubts crept in, and the labyrinth felt overwhelming. But hey, we all have those days right?

I clung to the memories of those hard-fought victories from the first time. They were my lifeline and all I had, a reminder that I had faced the abyss before and had clawed my way back. I had to believe I could do it again, that my spirit was stronger than this.

Yet something was different. I could not shake the discouragement quite so easily this time. When I did leave my home to visit my rehab specialist Dr. Moses, the gravity of the situation became painfully clear.

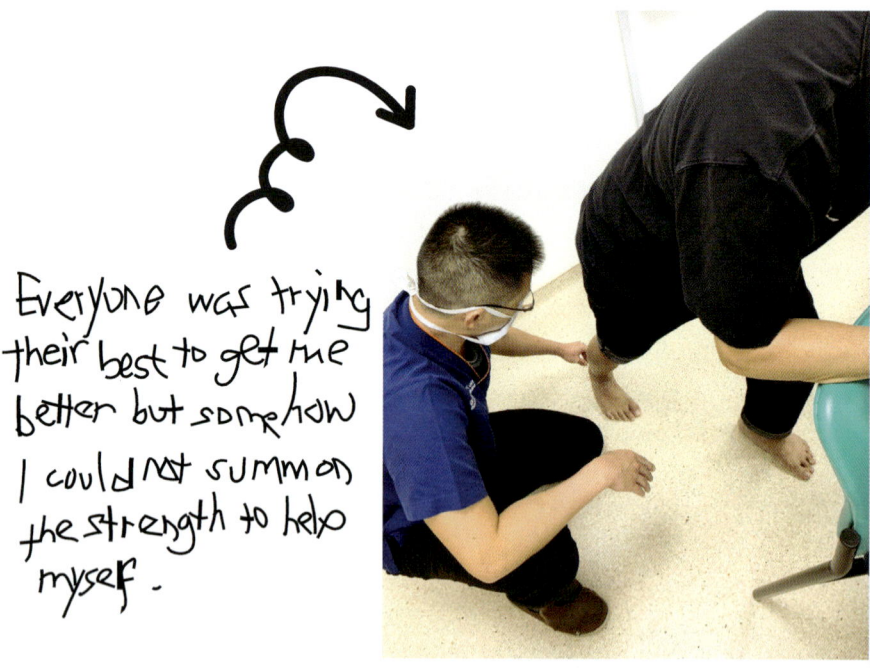

Everyone was trying their best to get me better but somehow I could not summon the strength to help myself.

"So, have you made an appointment with the physiotherapist I asked you to see?" Dr. Moses, with his characteristic warmth, began our conversation. My hesitation, a persistent habit of putting things off, lingered in the silence. "Next time, soon…" It was a reflexive promise that I had grown accustomed to making. I knew I had to do something, but I was not sure I would ever get around to it.

The days crawled along, interspersed with the usual sessions of occupational therapy. After months of not leaving my home, my concerned occupational therapist, Sijie, could not watch on anymore. He refused to let me surrender to defeat, and told me we were going to try something different.

With a gentle but firm approach, Sijie pointed me outside my home. It was terrifying; I felt like I was walking into a giant obstacle course waiting to consume me whole. Sijie, sensing my unease, adjusted his pace to match mine. He walked slowly beside me, offering silent support as I tried to navigate my neighbourhood.

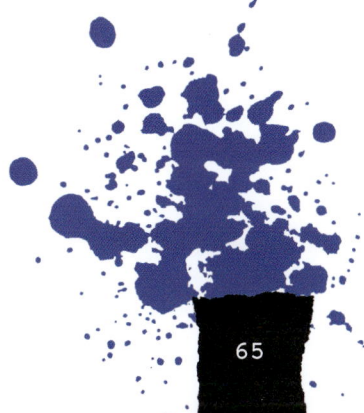

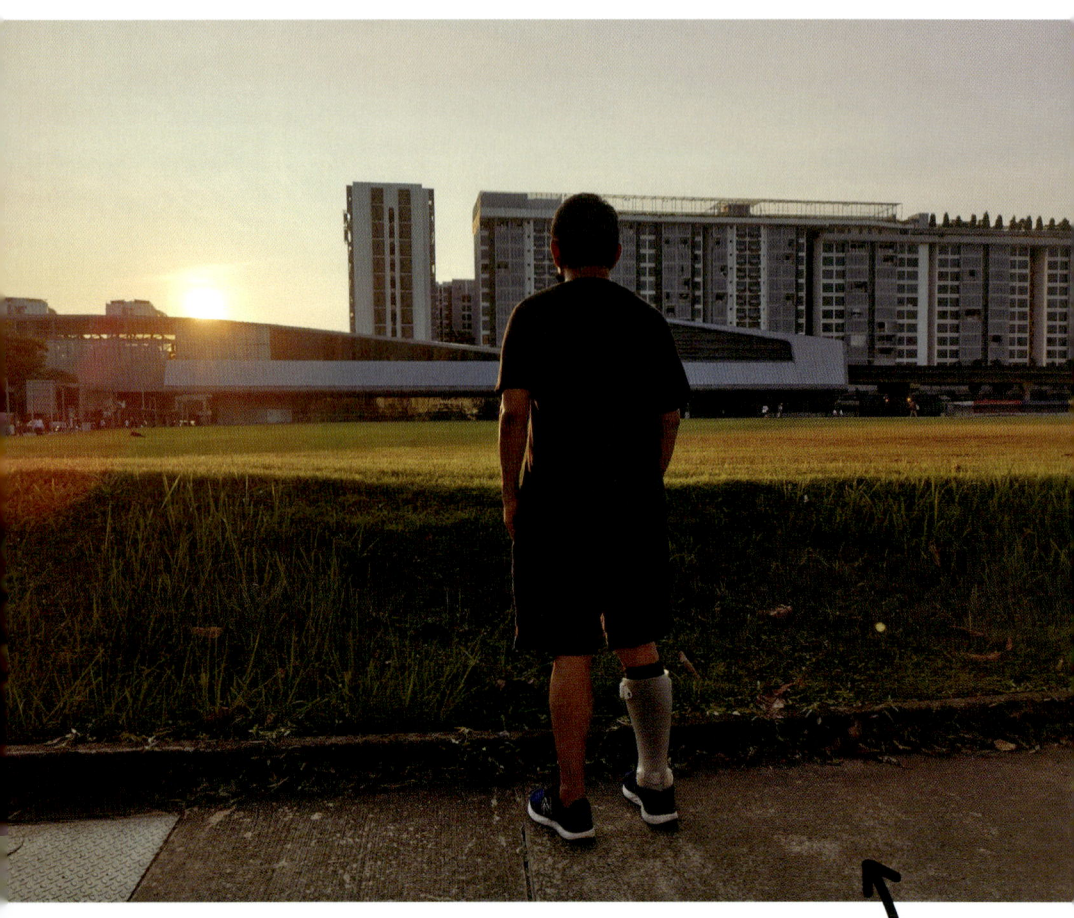

Rediscovering the beauty I had overlooked. Sometimes it is in the moments we have missed that we truly find gratitude.

I was not sure what I was expecting, but as I summoned the courage to venture forth, it was like a part of me was awakening. With each step, the warm sunshine and breeze brought the scent of freshly cut grass, filling my lungs with renewal. And the once intimidating figures gradually morphed into kind faces of encouragement.

The anxiety eventually dissipated, making way for a new appreciation. It was a strange sensation I had not experienced in a long time — hope. Contrary to my initial apprehension, it was not that bad after all. I found myself smiling, like I was getting ready to face the world again. And the world, with arms wide open, could not have given me a warmer welcome.

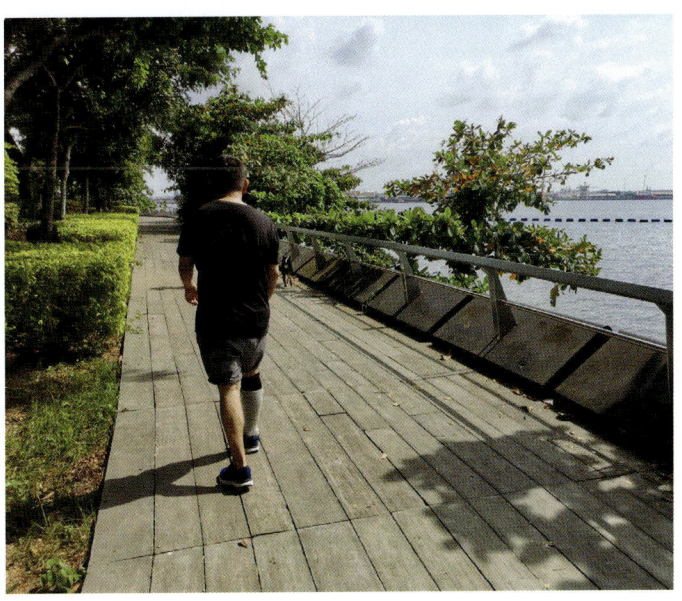

"Paint your story in colours as vibrant as you are!"

— Joey Lee

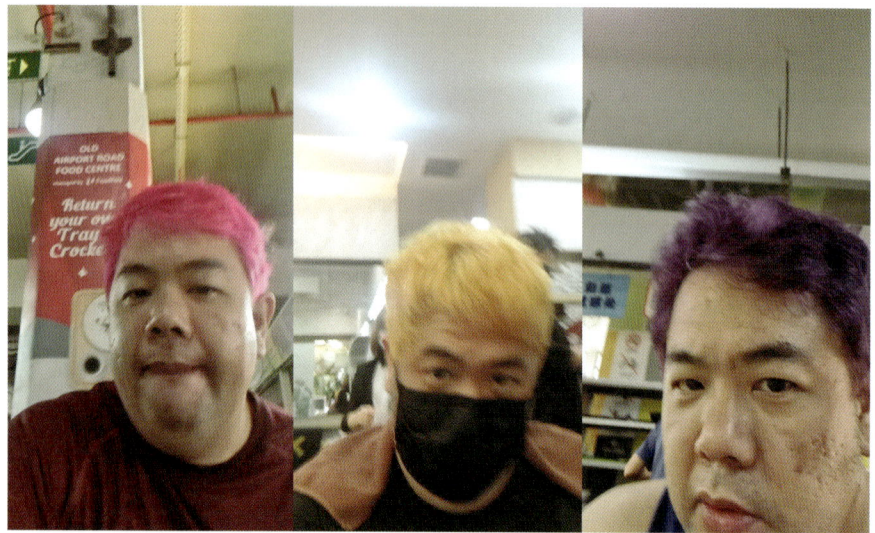

Life was humming along, with money flowing
in from my limousine business, a venture I
had built from the ground up. But my world,
once filled with the buzz of business
deals and the purr of luxury cars, took
a 180-degree turn after the stroke that
almost claimed my life.

One of my blood vessels had burst; I was lying on the hospital bed, unconscious and on the edge of death. The doctors told my wife they would have to pull the life support plug if I did not wake up within 24 hours. Everything was hanging in the balance.

Miraculously, I did. As I opened my eyes to the faces of those I loved, I knew I had been given a second chance. Pain was a constant companion, but the support of my family, especially my wife, kept me grounded. She stepped into the role of caretaker, shouldering the responsibilities that once were shared. She was truly the glue holding my family together.

I counted myself amongst the fortunate by being able to afford therapy even if it was just a weekly occurrence. I knew it was going to be crucial, especially in the first year following the stroke. My muscles were contracting due to inactivity, and the limbs on my affected side had begun to shrink.

So I threw myself into the process, motivated by the desire never to be bound again by the confines of a hospital bed. Being a type 2 diabetic also added an extra layer of urgency. I made myself walk and climb steps every day, even if only for 15 to 20 minutes. To my surprise, my legs regained strength at a much faster pace than I expected.

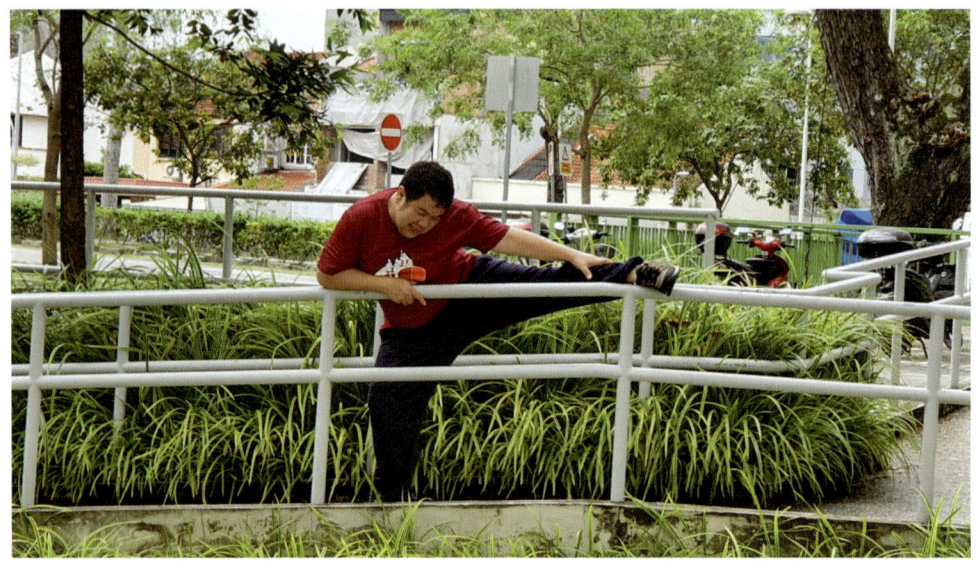

I wanted to push myself harder to get back to my pre-stroke state. In a way, the most challenging bit was learning to gauge my limits and listen to my body. It was only in knowing when to slow down that I found comfort in changing lifestyle habits and appreciating the simpler things.

Although I took everything in stride, I never stopped. I wanted others to know that having a stroke did not mean life was over. It is the fear of pain that often holds people back from the hard work of recovery. I even started a YouTube channel to share my journey. The year 2020, marked by global reckoning and COVID-19, became a year of personal transformation for me.

That was when I also transitioned into becoming a full-time Gojek driver. This shift allowed me to redefine success. Happiness, I realised, was not something to be purchased. It could be as simple as understanding what my body needed versus what I wanted.

While my days of selling limousines may be in the past, my present is now dedicated to a new purpose — charity work and helping others, just as so many have done for me. There is something really fulfilling about turning what happened to me into something positive. I hope to continue advocating for stroke awareness and building a community that stands together against the challenges we face.

NEW FRIENDS

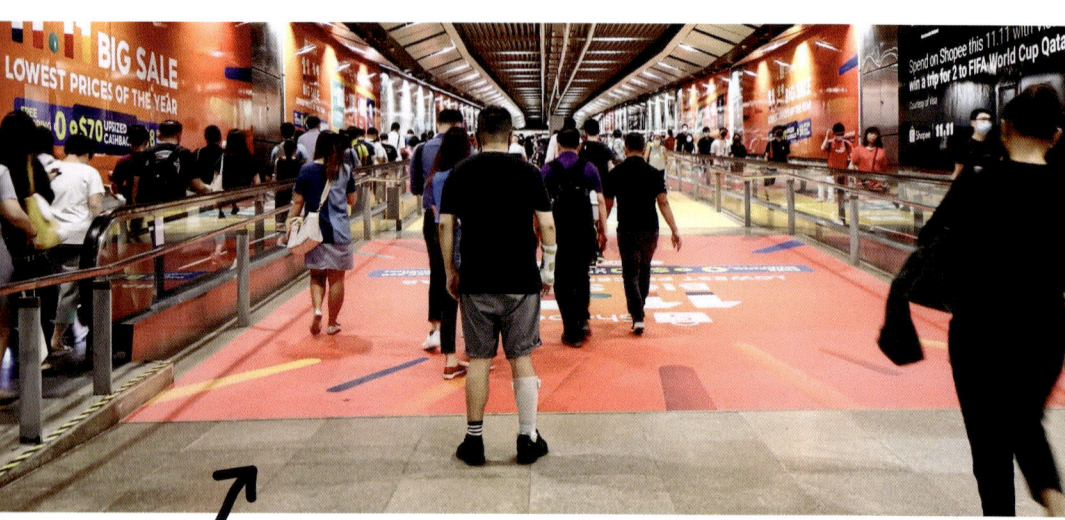

Just constantly feeling wiped out.
Talking these days is like running a
marathon, too tired to chat -

Despite my valiant efforts, social interaction with friends and family was often an area that proved challenging. Their genuine concern, although appreciated, does come with the wearisome task of having to explain what happened to me or what I needed, especially with aphasia affecting my speech and memory.

It was serendipitous that I would then find connection within the support groups and members from Singapore National Stroke Association and Aphasia SG. At first, I was happy to just listen in and let others lead the conversation. But as we got talking, I found there was a lot I wanted to say.

Here in these groups of survivors, I was met with more than just shared experiences; there was understanding and empathy. It was a judgement-free circle where I could be open about my struggles without worrying about being misunderstood.

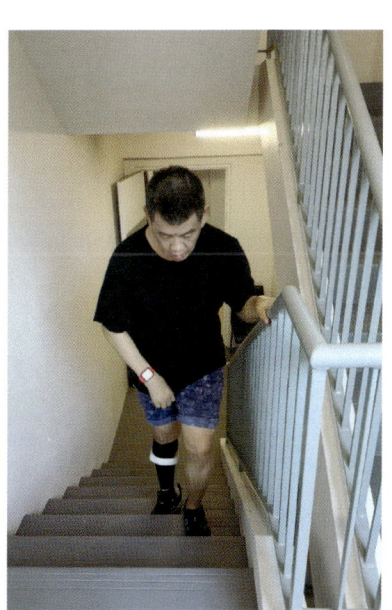

Terence (T): "As much as I want to stay positive, there are moments where I feel overwhelmed. I keep thinking, what more is there after this? The fear of having another stroke and new complications is also always on my mind."

Joey (J): "I know what you mean… I've been down this road as well. For me, reflecting on where I started versus where I am now helps. I remember those early days in the hospital and how far I've come since then. I use that to motivate myself, to never return to the hospital bed again."

T: "But I think what's most frustrating is the fact that progress can be so slow. It's hard to be patient and keep faith, especially when you're used to being on the move and achieving things."

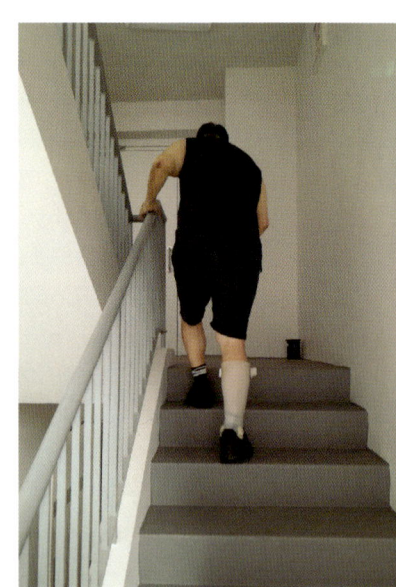

J: "That's why it helps to have people who understand. We're here, having this conversation, supporting each other. That itself is a significant achievement. We're not alone in this battle."

I did not get all the answers I wanted, but still, it made a big difference. It was a breath of fresh air that focused my energy away from the swirling questions, and towards more constructive ends. I had to find a way to move forward. It was time to pull myself together and rebuild my life.

While it did not seem like it at the time, I can see now that the fall had been a blessing in disguise. It was the sign I needed to slow down, and fortunately, I came out on the other side pretty much intact. My new friends have shown me that while hitting rock bottom has its share of difficulties, there is always a chance at redemption.

Little by little, I found my footing and returned to the world that once seemed so far away. This time, I no longer felt like I was in the shadows — I was going to put myself out there and take charge of my story again. Most of all, I was proud that I had fallen, and I had gotten back up.

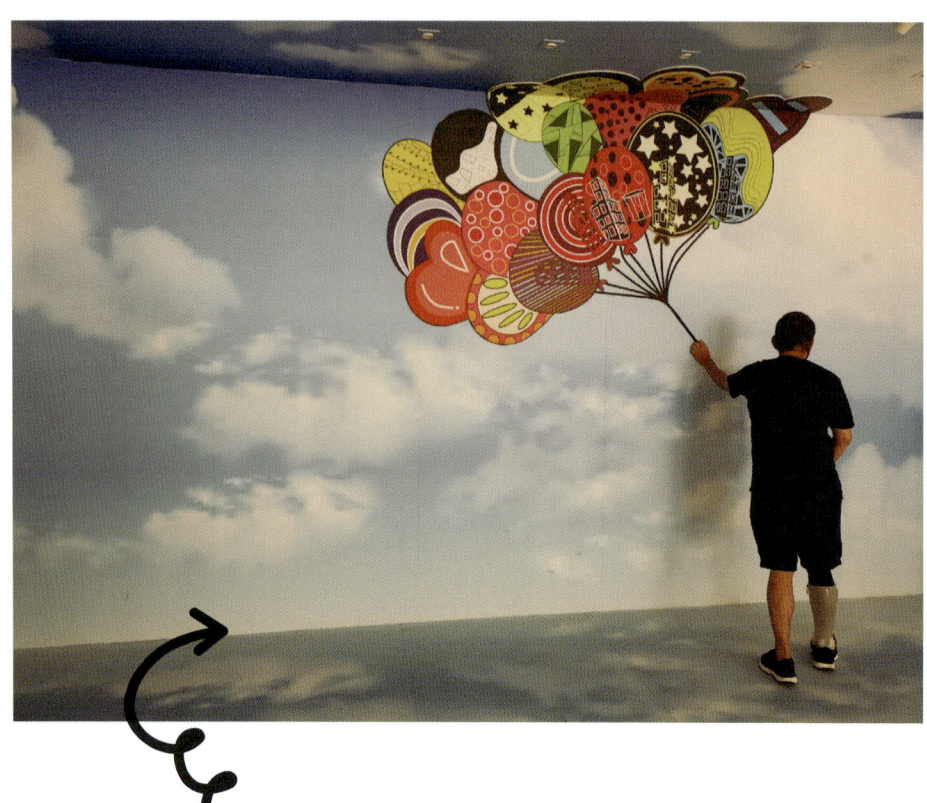

There is strength in vulnerability and
when you have hit rock bottom,
the only way is up!

"I turned stroke into a chance to become a better version of myself."

— Alvin Chee

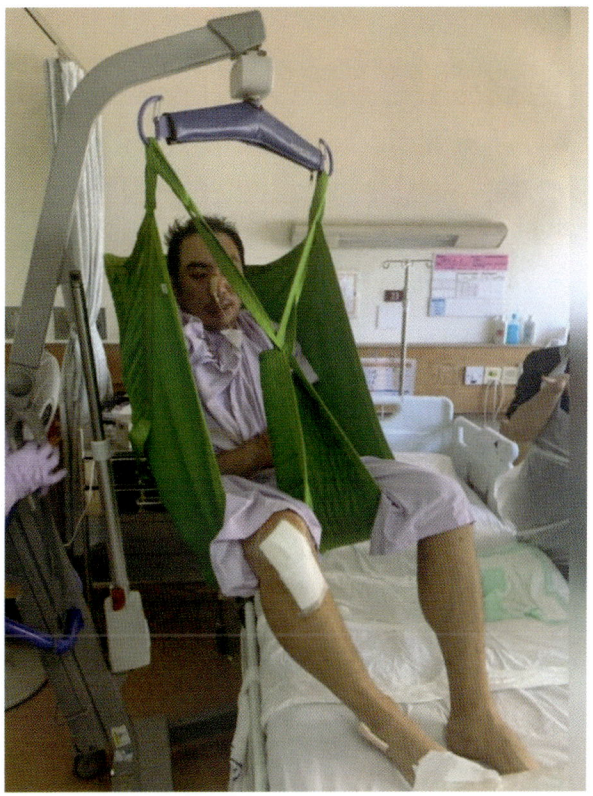

In 2021, my life altered drastically when I suffered a stroke. Two months of rehab therapy at Tan Tock Seng Hospital passed before I could even walk again.

Tasks as basic as bathing posed challenges, and I often felt helpless. But I refused to surrender, knowing that recovery is different for everyone and each stroke survivor has their own unique timeline. Some may take a shorter time, while others require longer periods of dedication.

Before the stroke, I was a housing agent, and work took up most of my time. I used to smoke and drink a lot. My exercise routine was sporadic at best — the occasional run, but nothing too consistent. After the stroke, I realised that I needed to make changes to my lifestyle.

Emerging from that challenging period, I decided that my journey was also going to be one of transformation. I decided to become someone new, someone better. I became Alvin, the guy who loves fitness and does not back down from a challenge.

I started going for therapy at the Stroke Support Station (S3), gradually easing back into work. This was followed by yoga and gym sessions at ActiveSG. Although the first months were tough, exercise eventually became a kind of haven, with physical therapy playing a crucial role in helping me get back on my feet.

Through dedicated efforts and a personalised stretching package, I progressed from struggling to even sit on the floor to achieving the ability to kneel down. My goal was not just to regain my physical abilities but also to become more independent like I used to be.

While subsidies made therapy more accessible, it was still quite an expensive endeavour. Fortunately, a social worker stepped in to help with the money stuff. This caring person guided me along the process, making sure I had all the support I needed. Recognising the emotional toll financial stress can take, their help ensured I could focus on healing without the added pressure.

My friends and wife took turns driving me to therapy, ferrying me through those tough times. Thankfully, I had friends who also had strokes, and we helped each other out a lot along the way. The stroke community became a source of support, gathering at coffee shops to share tips, experiences, and words of encouragement.

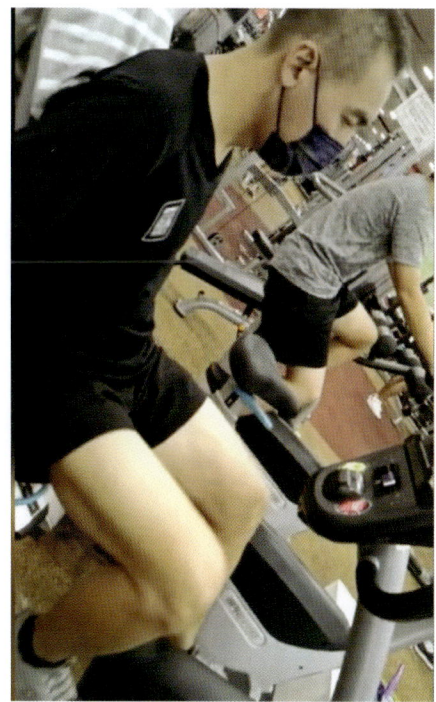

Through it all, I have been lucky enough to turn a tough situation into a chance to become stronger. My story shows that we can handle hardships, overcome problems, and not just survive but do well. Facing challenges can be turned into stepping stones for personal growth, helping us become a better, more powerful version of ourselves.

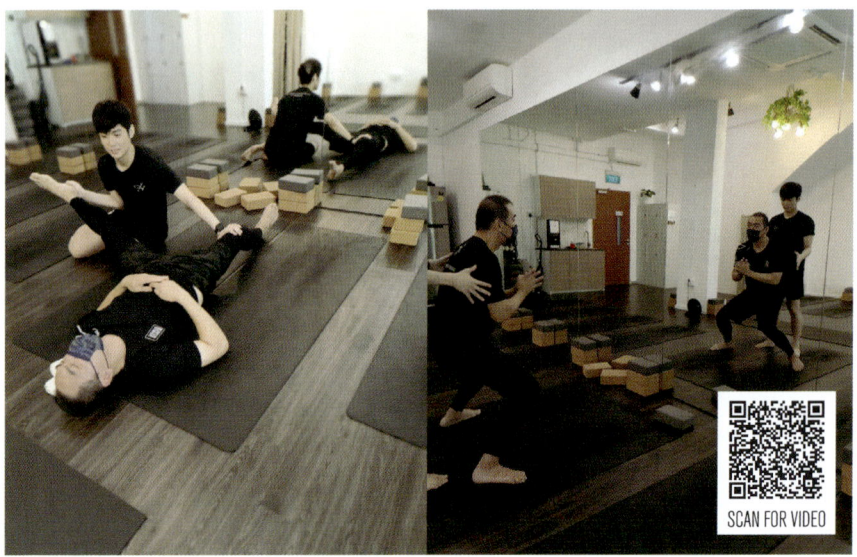

SCAN FOR VIDEO

TAKING THE BRACE OFF

Daily rituals of strapping on braces and leaning on canes had become a part of my identity, almost an extension of who I was. Now, in the absence of those confining devices, it felt strangely bittersweet.

It was Dr. Moses who really pushed me to get back to physiotherapy after my fall. I have to admit that my initial enthusiasm was lacking, having largely fallen behind from inactivity. My muscles were weak and like rocks, and mostly, I was afraid I would not be able to keep up with the exercises. I was sure I would end up disappointing Dr. Moses, but him being a constant voice of reason, urged that it was a necessary step for my recovery. I had to put in the work if I wanted to see progress.

So I gritted my teeth and went along. Yan Fen, my recently assigned physiotherapist, entered my life with a pragmatic approach, showing a sharp awareness of the physical hurdles I faced. Our efforts took shape in a comprehensive strategy aimed at tackling my challenges comprehensively. The experience proved to be far from pleasant — it was a mix of pain, frustration, and a great amount of perspiration.

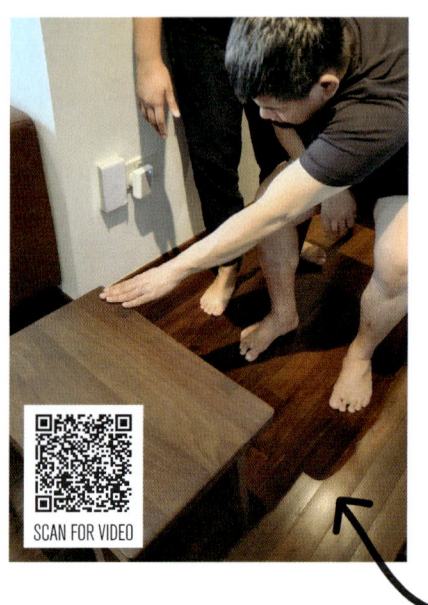

SCAN FOR VIDEO

The initial sessions were anything but easy - if I thought OT was hard, physio was a rude awakening.

I found myself grimacing and contorting as Yan Fen applied a range of techniques — pushing, pulling, and whatever it took to get my muscles moving again. I had underestimated the challenge and had no idea my body could protest so much against movement. Each attempt to regain mobility was met with significant internal protest. I was hot, tired, and constantly in pain.

Yan Fen, though, is a champ dealing with my whining, and she deserves a medal for it. I knew I was a difficult patient, but she never made me feel like a burden. Every time I felt like giving up, she would point out some tiny improvement. She would say, her smile contagious, "See, you're getting better!" or "Hey, you lifted your leg a bit higher today!", elevating what seemed like a trivial achievement into a noteworthy triumph.

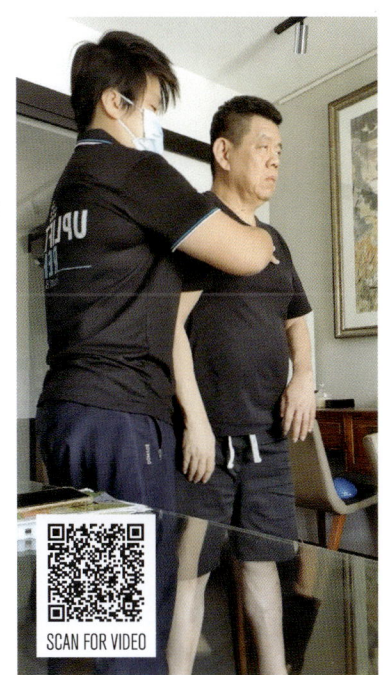

SCAN FOR VIDEO

The initial discomfort did not magically disappear, but there was a peculiar satisfaction in the pain. It was the kind that told me something was shifting beneath the surface, like my body was shooting me a message — a kind of "things are happening here" sort of vibe.

Yan Fen, with her unique blend of professionalism and empathy, illuminated the path forward by recounting the triumphs of her other patients, showing that progress was definitely within reach. And I also learnt that physiotherapy is not just a one-way street focused on recovery. It can also serve to prevent injuries.

Balance, especially, is a critical component that affects me. It is important, as it reduces the risk of falls, one of the most common challenges faced by stroke survivors. The balance exercises Yan Fen prescribed not only enhanced my physical capabilities but also contributed to rebuilding my confidence in moving safely.

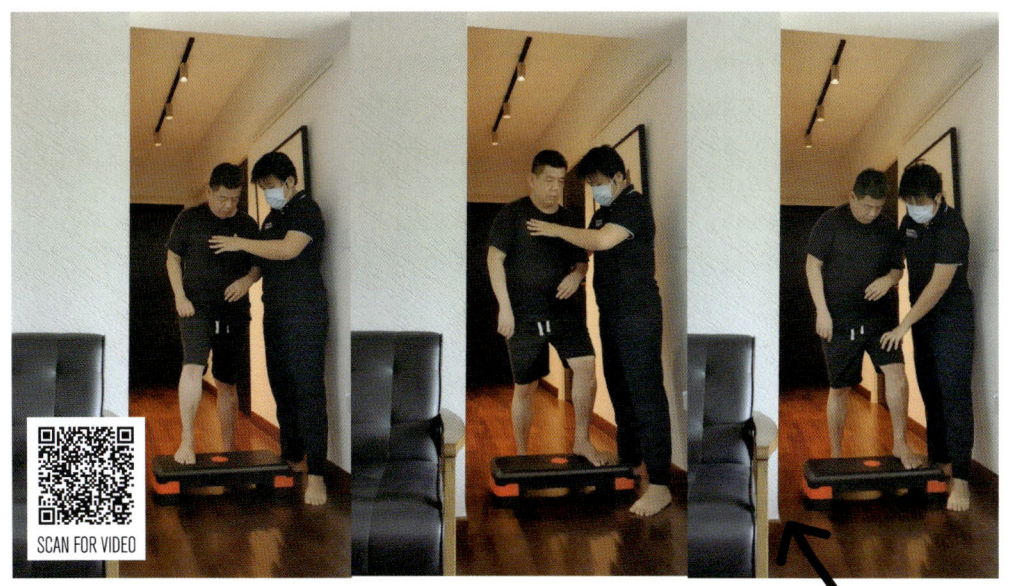

SCAN FOR VIDEO

Breaking up with laziness and getting cosy with exercise... the end result — feeling way better!

Acknowledging the brain's tendency to forget learned movements, homework assignments became another part of my routine — exercises and activities to be practised daily in the comfort of my home. At first, I was hesitant. I did not want to add more tasks to my already busy schedule. But Yan Fen assured me that this consistent practice would help reinforce the skills I had learned and make them an integral part of my muscle memory.

As I started incorporating these tasks into my daily routine, I realised that they were not as time-consuming as I had anticipated. Yan Fen had designed them in a way that they could easily be done in short intervals throughout the day. I also found that I was able to do them at my own pace, without any pressure.

Eventually, weeks turned into months, and it seemed my brain had finally accepted these tasks as part of my routine, making them easier to remember and complete. My muscles automatically knew what to do, and I could feel myself becoming stronger and more coordinated. It became a form of self-care, and I looked forward to it every day.

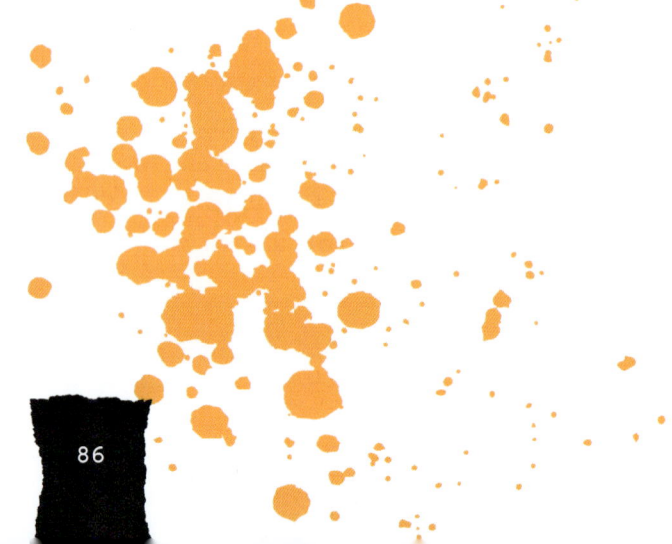

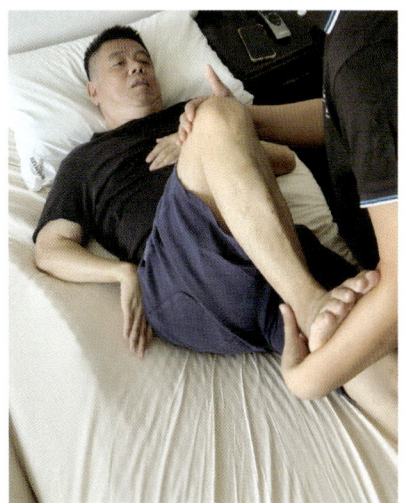

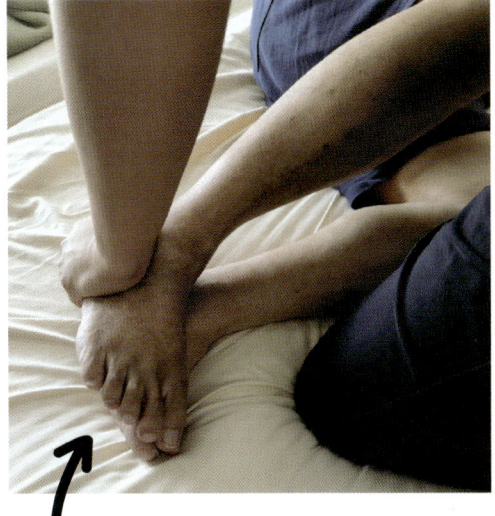

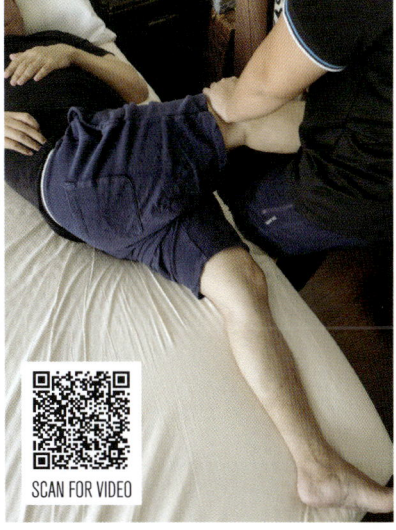

SCAN FOR VIDEO

There is something cool about how the most unglamorous routine can quietly turn into a roadmap for getting stronger and more put together.

"Many people think physio-therapists just do massages but that is not true."

— Koh Yan Fen

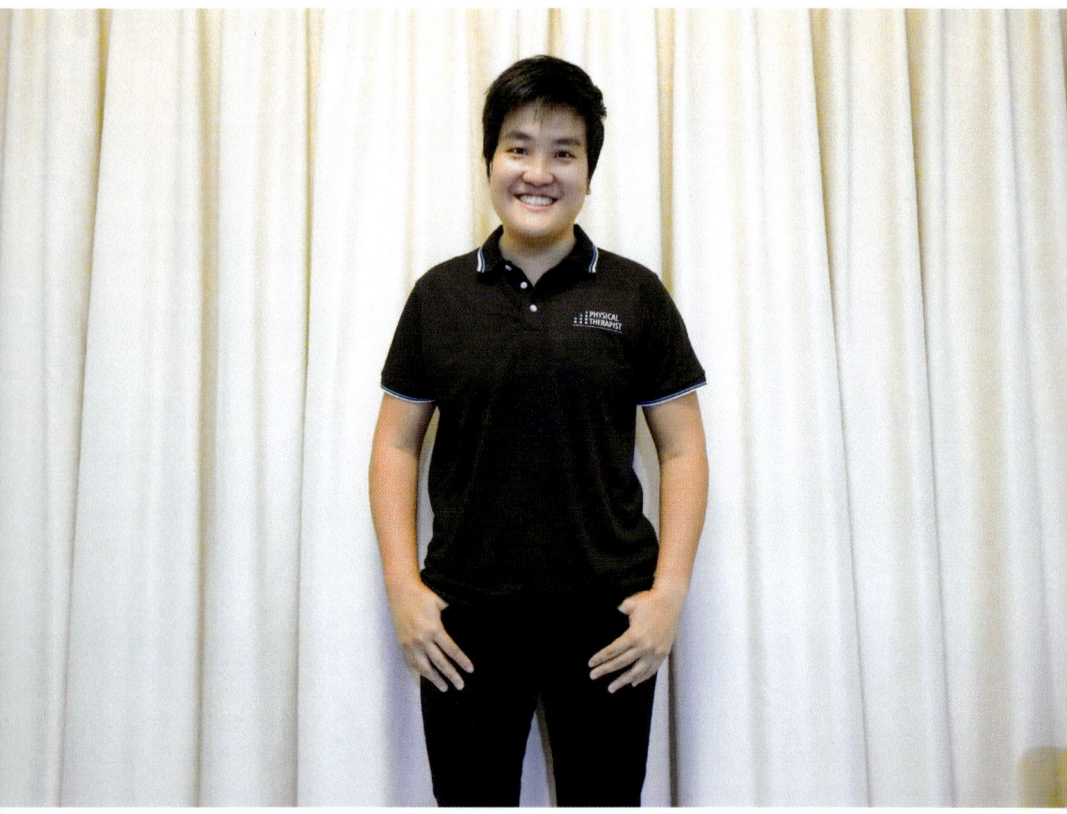

Choosing the path of a physiotherapist
specialising in neurological conditions
like strokes and Parkinson's disease was a
deliberate and meaningful decision for me.
It all began when my grandmother was admitted

to the hospital, and I witnessed firsthand the interactions and dynamics between healthcare professionals and patients.

My grandmother suffered from a blood disorder, and her bone marrow failed to produce enough blood cells. She spent many years in and out of the hospital until her eventual passing. The experience ignited a curiosity to delve deeper into this field and explore ways to assist individuals facing such challenges.

While some might think physiotherapists are akin to masseuses, the reality is quite different. Being a physiotherapist involves completing a comprehensive four-year university education to acquire a degree qualification and another two years of work supervision to obtain a full licence under the Allied Health Professions Council (AHPC) to practise in Singapore.

Following this foundation, extensive years of dedicated work and experience allow us to specialise in areas such as Orthopedics, Neurology, Cardiorespiratory, Pediatrics, Geriatrics, Sports, Women's Health, and more. These specialised focuses equip us with in-depth knowledge and expertise to address diverse health conditions and unique patient needs.

When it comes to strokes, physiotherapists play a critical role in the immediate aftermath. Neuroplasticity, early mobilisation, and early rehabilitation have been shown to be beneficial for motor recovery after a stroke. Therefore, it is important to commence therapy promptly after the first day of the stroke, with the primary goal of optimising outcomes.

The initial weeks are the most challenging as the brain has lost significant function, and patients are heavily dependent on therapists' assistance to move. Physiotherapists in the acute setting focus on aiding them with movement in their affected limbs, assisting them in regaining mobility, and preventing complications like muscle stiffness or contractures that may arise from prolonged immobility.

Beyond the acute phase, physiotherapists in the community ensure a seamless transition and provide tailored rehabilitation plans focused on individual needs and goals. These personal goals encompass a wide spectrum, ranging from a desire to return to work post-stroke, re-engaging in activities they used to enjoy, like gardening and cooking, or simply reclaiming roles such as parenting, playing and bonding with their children.

Achieving these goals involves an extensive journey of rehabilitation and dedication from our patients. Along the way, we celebrate every small success with them, recognising that each milestone signifies a step forward in their journey towards recovery.

As a home-based physiotherapist, I consider myself part of a team alongside my patients, working together towards their return to normal life after injury or illness. My primary focus revolves around helping my patients regain physical abilities that we often do not think about when we are healthy — simple things like standing, walking, and doing daily tasks. By carefully assessing how my patients move or struggle to move, be it issues with strength, balance,

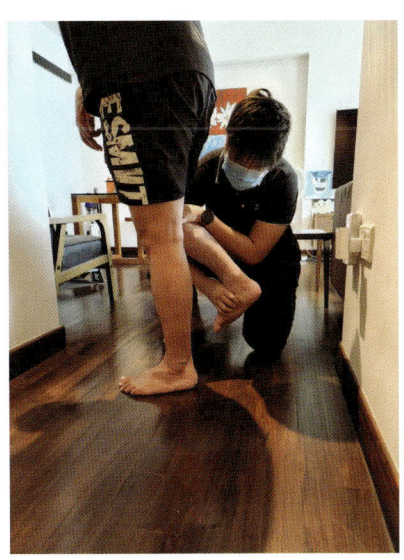
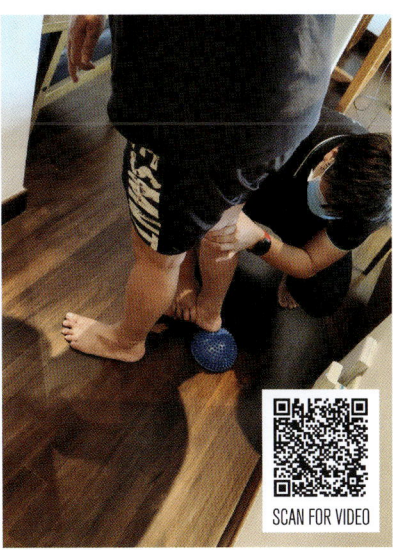

SCAN FOR VIDEO

coordination, etc., identifying the root cause of these limitations is important for an effective targeted treatment.

I firmly believe in tailoring treatments uniquely to each individual, ensuring that our interventions precisely target what they need to improve and make everyday activities easier for them. Collaborating closely with patients and other healthcare professionals, our goal is not just physical recovery but also empowering individuals to reclaim their passions and embrace a fulfilling life.

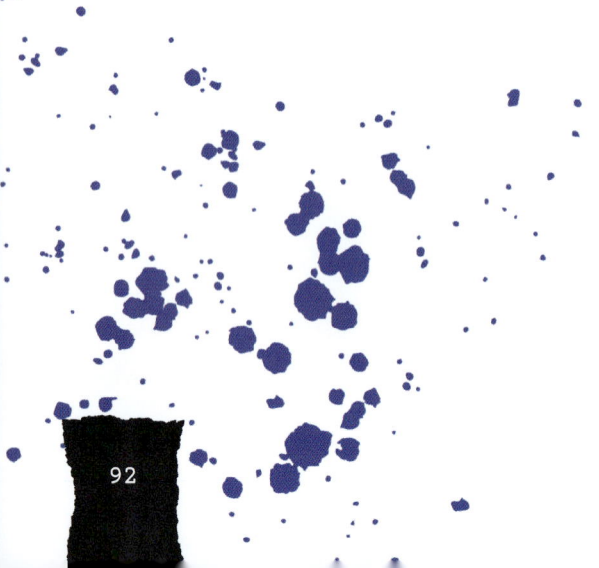

"Physical therapy is the cornerstone of stroke rehabilitation."

— Dr. Moses Koh

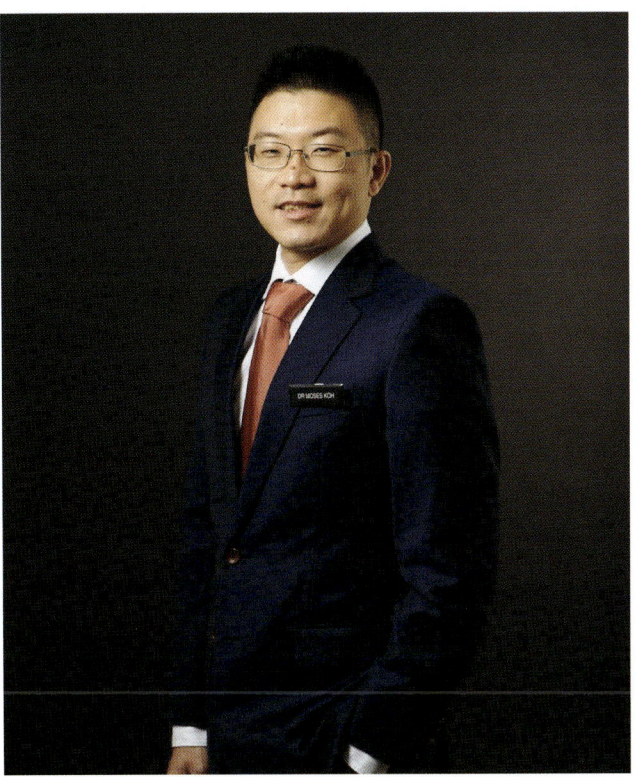

At the conclusion of his first book, hope permeated the story of Terence, a resilient stroke survivor. However, life's journey proved more tumultuous than anticipated. In September 2022, a fall left Terence with a fractured right wrist, compelling him to begin his recovery anew.

Witnessing Terence's journey firsthand, I understand the impact a fall or an unexpected event can have on a patient's confidence and progress. Ambulation became a challenge once more, and occupational therapy for his right upper limb was abruptly paused. It was a daunting setback, disrupting the semblance of progress he had painstakingly made.

The journey of recovery after a stroke is multifaceted, so let me share some fundamental guiding principles utilised in physical therapy for neurorehabilitation.

The Forced Use Paradigm or Learned "non-use" underscores the importance of compelling the use of affected parts, preventing the tendency to neglect them. Exercise quality forms a cornerstone, and Terence's story is a good illustration of how therapy does that.

Repetitive, intense, goal-oriented, functional, massed, and active routines facilitate neural repair, and have helped Terence the most in regaining his stability and ability to walk again and improving his upper limb function. Another remarkable phenomenon is Cross-modal Plasticity, which involves employing unaffected systems to compensate for those affected by the stroke, tapping into the brain's innate capacity for adaptation and recovery.

Optimal learning necessitates feedback
mechanisms encompassing visual, auditory,
and tactile signals, accelerating
the learning process. And while early
intervention maximises neuroplasticity,
capitalising on the brain's adaptive
potential for better outcomes, the journey
is far from over.

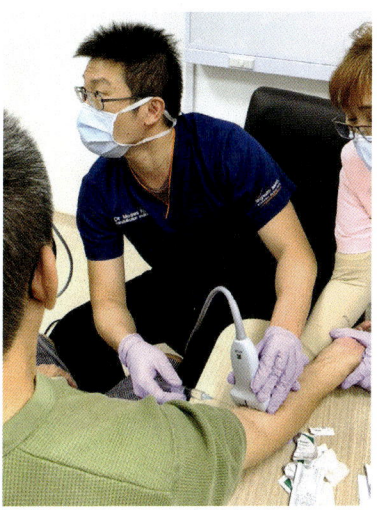

The misconception that the golden period
concludes after six months is a pitfall that
some often succumb to. The reality is that
while the initial surge of recovery may
plateau, I have seen patients continue to
make progress over time.

It takes a sustained effort and commitment
towards maintaining and achieving a certain
level of physical function that extends
beyond those first months. For stroke

patients, the challenges they face are even more complex, as the ageing process also poses another obstacle, with the body naturally inclining towards decline.

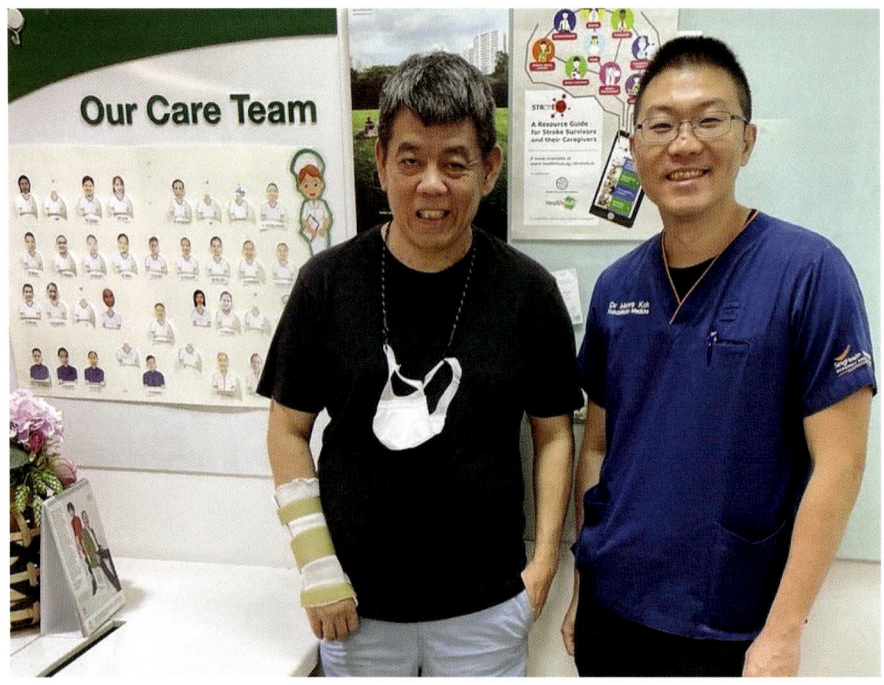

Enriching the rehabilitation environment is therefore crucial, and family, social support, and peer encouragement play an invaluable role in fostering progress and rebuilding lives. The principles of neurorehabilitation serve as guiding lights in the arduous yet hopeful journey of individuals like Terence, navigating the complexities of stroke recovery.

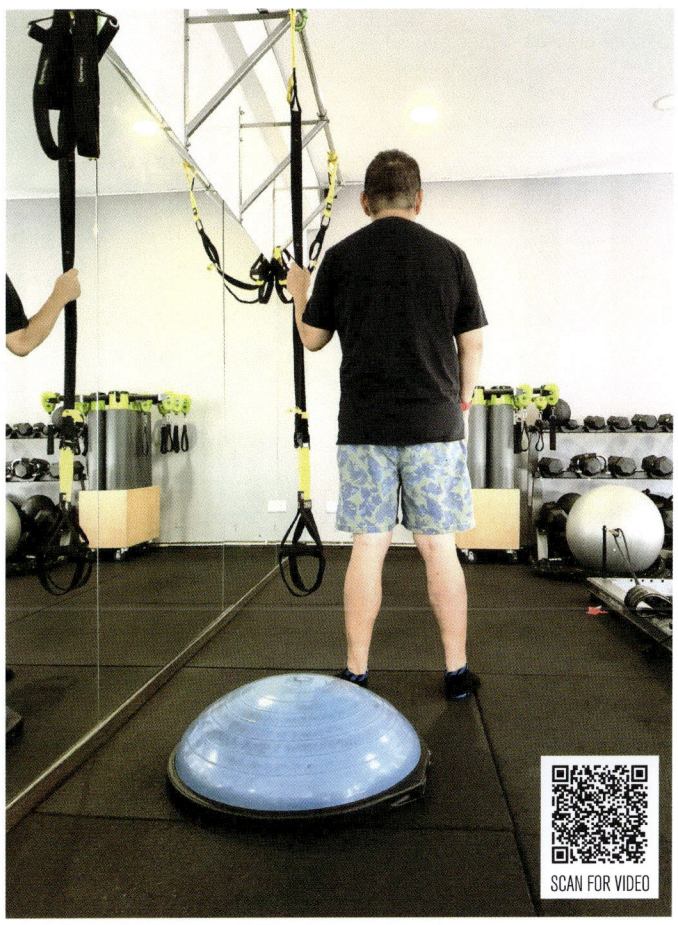

SCAN FOR VIDEO

In my 20s, I stumbled upon Pilates but dismissed it as a luxury reserved for the rich and famous. The few classes I tried did not capture my interest, and I found them rather dull and monotonous. Fast forward to the age of 58 — and life took an unexpected turn with my stroke three years ago.

Stroke survivors like me face an uphill battle. The brain, that magnificent control centre of the body, suddenly becomes a complex puzzle, and one finds themselves battling with a body that will not cooperate.

I threw myself into various forms of exercise, consulting occupational and physical therapists to guide my rehabilitation. I revisited the subject of Pilates, and initially, I could not fathom how a discipline developed by Joseph Pilates in the early 20th century could help me. But desperate for progress, I dove in.

That was when I met Ann, a Pilates instructor who changed my perception of the discipline. Entering a Pilates studio for the first time in decades, I was met with an array of strange-looking machines. They were intimidating, to say the least, but Ann's warm and reassuring smile put me at ease.

As we started with the basic Pilates exercises, I could not help but marvel at how deceptively challenging they were. Every move was a calculated effort, my muscles protesting like disgruntled employees in a Monday morning meeting. As the class progressed, we moved through a series of exercises that worked not only my core but also my arms, legs, and back. I could feel my muscles working hard.

Ann's patience and expertise became evident as she adjusted the exercises to accommodate my physical limitations. One vivid moment I remember was when she adjusted the straps to accommodate my arm's limited range of motion. It was a small change, but it made a world of difference in my ability to engage in the exercise effectively.

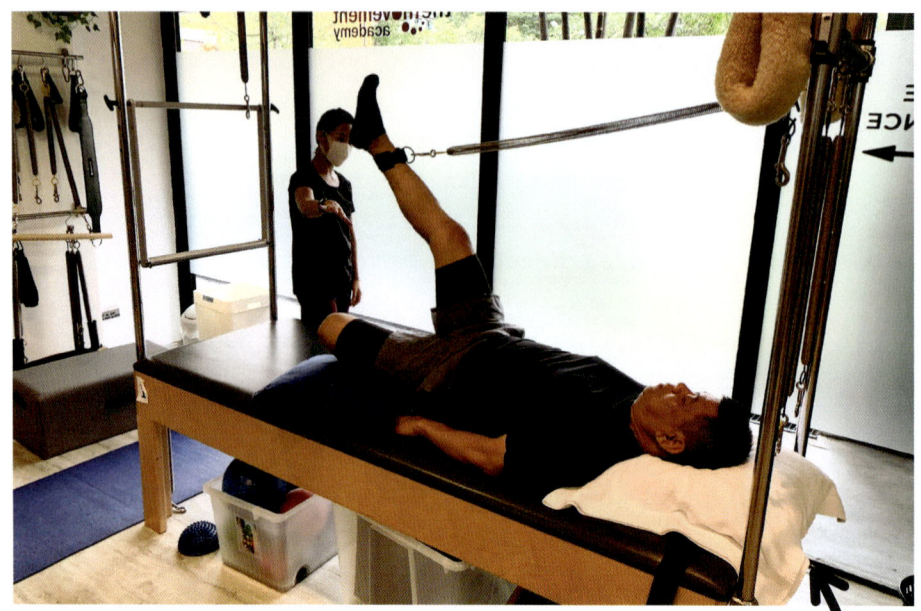

We all could do with a good stretch — in fact, you probably need one right now!

So I continued to return for Pilates sessions. My right muscles were especially weak, so we worked on them to see if they could provide some support. Ann's ability to recognise when a movement was not working for me spoke volumes to her expertise. She never hesitated to suggest alternatives if I could not feel a particular movement or if it was causing discomfort. Ever resourceful, she would gently guide me toward an alternative.

In the midst of a session, if a movement felt unfamiliar or confusing, Ann would encourage me to look at my reflection in the mirror. It was a reminder that sometimes, the visual can offer clarity when our proprioceptive senses falter. And it was while we were executing a particularly challenging stretch that Ann's keen eyes captured my extra effort when I knew a camera was focused on me.

Low lunges exercises encourage my right calf muscles to be concentrically contracted, with resistance for strengthening. Ankle mobility work is happening as well.

SCAN FOR VIDEO

Observing how I became more attuned to my movements and more conscious of my posture, Ann's suggestion to document my Pilates journey through photos was kind of ingenious in boosting my participation. Her strategy brought a new level of conscientiousness to my approach. It was no longer just about going through the motions; I had to make every movement count.

I grumbled when I saw pictures where I did not look as graceful as I wished to be. I felt accountable to the lens, compelled to give my best in every moment. This served me well, on one hand to look good in photos, but on the other hand, to also prove to myself that I could rise above my challenges.

Activities such as chest openers were aimed at reducing tightness, promoting better body posture, and even relieving upper back pain.

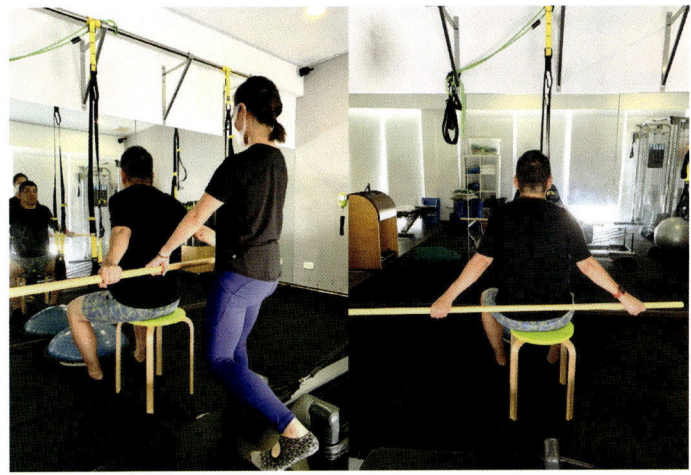

Sometimes, Ann expressed her concern that many people only seem to start exercising when something bad happens to their health. I nodded along; people tend to avoid exercise because they find it boring, just as I did when I thought about trying Pilates. But it should not take a life-altering event to appreciate its value.

Movement truly is a medicine that can heal not just the body but the spirit too. And Pilates, beginning as another physical rehabilitation tool, turned into something more – a holistic approach to my recovery. Each session built upon the last and fostered a heightened sense of body awareness, a mindfulness that extended into my everyday activities.

PiLATES ISN'T JUST FOR THE RICH AND FAMOUS

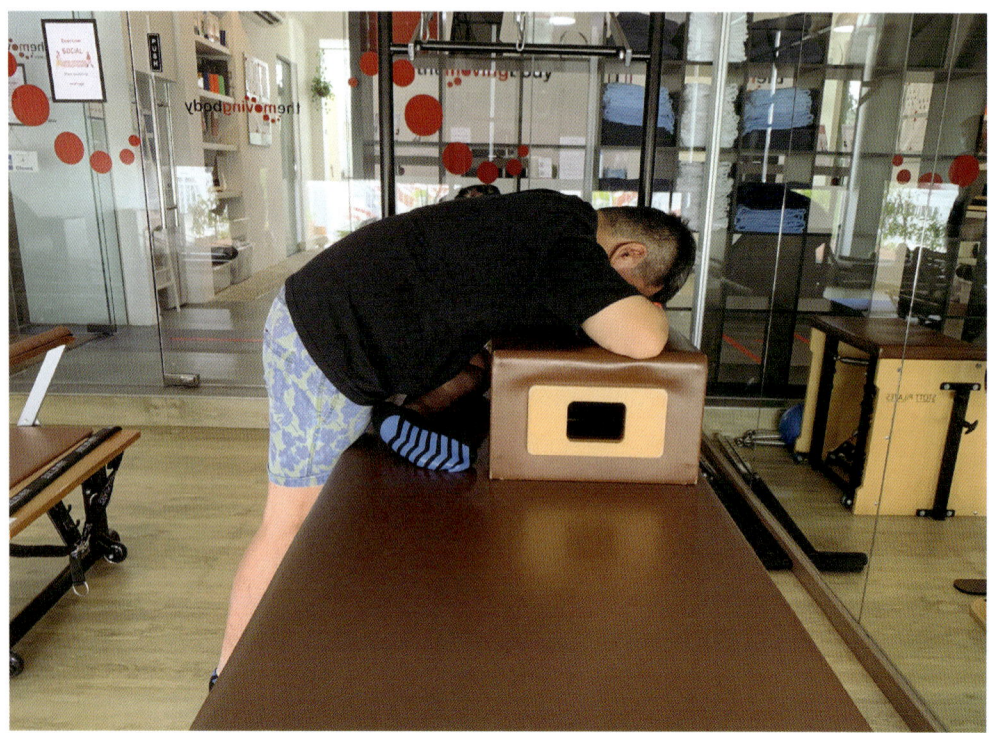

Pilates is a method of exercise that has a rich history spanning over a century. Initially, it gained popularity among professional dancers in the early 20th century as a means to prevent injuries and enhance flexibility. Today, it is a practice embraced by over 12 million individuals worldwide, but it is far more than just a passing fitness trend.

Supported by a wealth of historical significance and a growing body of scientific research, Pilates offers a myriad of physical and mental health benefits. Celebrities have also played a role in popularising the method, with Hollywood stars and public figures openly endorsing it and contributing to its mainstream appeal.

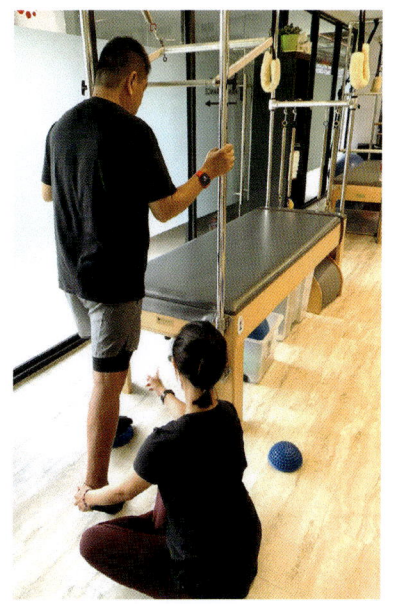

The practice has evolved to cater to a wide range of preferences, including classical Pilates, contemporary Pilates, and specialised approaches for different populations. Its adaptable nature allows it to be modified for individuals with varying needs and capabilities, and specialised Pilates programs have been developed for seniors, pregnant women, children, and individuals with disabilities. This inclusivity has made Pilates accessible to a broad demographic, not limited to any age group or fitness level.

Targeted workouts can help to improve mobility in various areas, which can become very limited in those with a sedentary lifestyle.

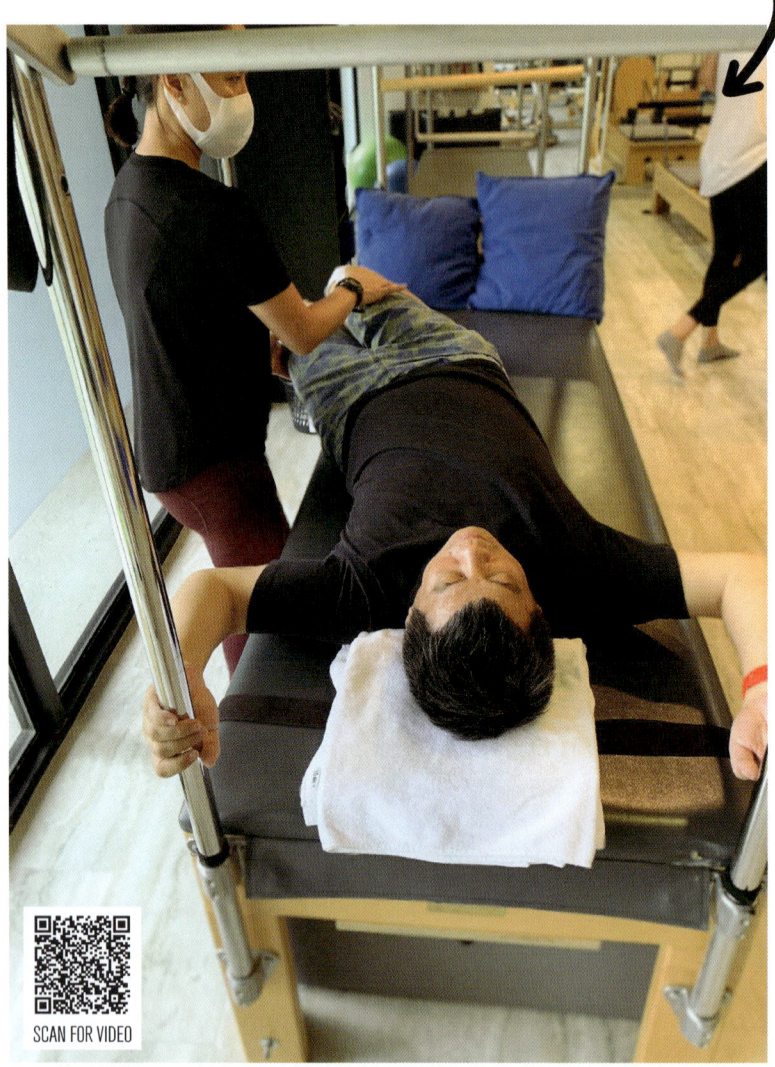

SCAN FOR VIDEO

In the world of Pilates, there is a great emphasis on the core. And while Pilates is often synonymous with building core strength, it also extends its reach to the muscles in the arms, back and legs. This comprehensive approach targets both the larger muscle groups and the smaller, stabilising muscles.

Research studies are validating its positive impact on areas such as back pain, postural alignment, and overall physical fitness, and many physical therapy practices now incorporate Pilates-based exercises into their rehabilitation programs. With its array of exercise modifications and equipment options that can intensify or decrease the challenge, Pilates is a versatile practice, allowing for a safe and effective workout for anyone and everyone.

In addition to its physical benefits, Pilates has also been recognised for its mental and emotional advantages. The mind-body connection fostered by the practice promotes relaxation, stress relief, and mindfulness. Many practitioners find that Pilates is not just a form of exercise but a holistic approach to well-being.

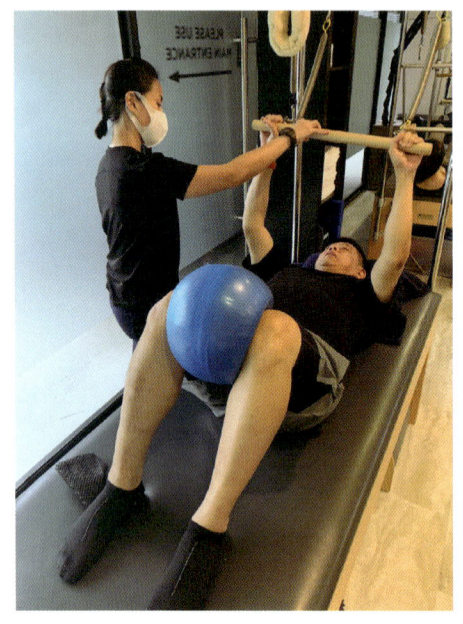

By squeezing the ball between my knees and ankles, I am enghging my adductors (inner thighs) and pelvic floor muscles (part of the core).

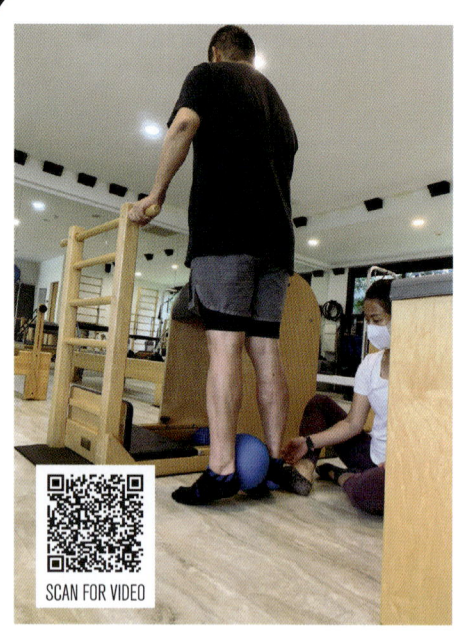

SCAN FOR VIDEO

"Get moving, energy creates energy!"

- Ann Ho

Ever since I was young, I have always been into movement and playing sports rather than following the usual academic paths.

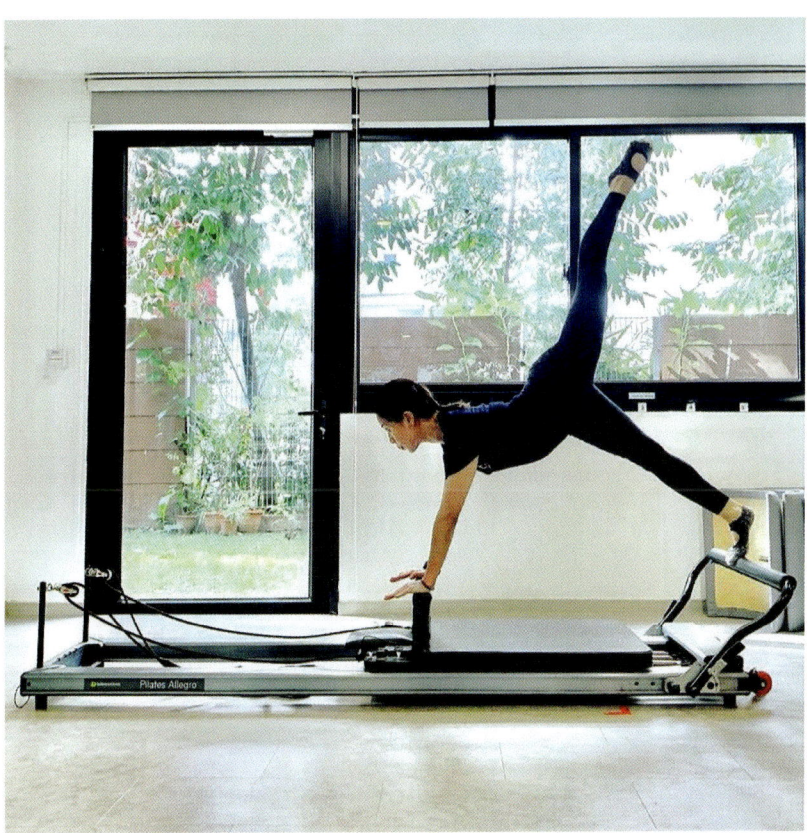

Initially setting my sights on a career as a yoga instructor, my plans changed due in part to my insightful mother-in-law. A seasoned Pilates instructor, she keenly noted the saturation in the yoga market, redirecting my focus toward Pilates.

Following her advice, I began exploring the world of Pilates and instantly knew I had found my true passion. What really hooked me was how Pilates focuses on exercises that are gentle on the body yet do wonders for mobility and strength. The gradual way it engages the core and fosters a deep connection with the body felt like a perfect fit for my own active lifestyle.

Eventually, I took the plunge and began teaching my own Pilates classes. It pushed me not only to grow in my role but also as an individual seeking to enhance their understanding of the human body. The real joy came from witnessing my students' progress and seeing their improved sense of well-being. It fuelled my determination to keep improving as an instructor.

It also became clear to me that even the most active person can face health crises. I distinctly remember those childhood moments watching my father effortlessly do push-ups; he was not just my inspiration but also my role model. He embodied the essence of an alpha male — constantly active and never shying away from pushing his limits. Yet he was forced to confront his health challenges when he suffered a stroke several years back.

I wanted to introduce my father to Pilates, and at first, he resisted the idea, perhaps out of pride or fear. But gradually, he began to understand the benefits. I knew once he started, he would appreciate it and participate more. I especially related to Terence's journey as well due to witnessing my father go through a stroke.

As Terence's pilates instructor, I found myself navigating a fine balance between encouraging him to push beyond his comfort zone and allowing him space to rest and recover. There were days when motivation seemed to elude him, and he would struggle with a sense of laziness. It was about understanding the right timing and knowing precisely when to push him a little further.

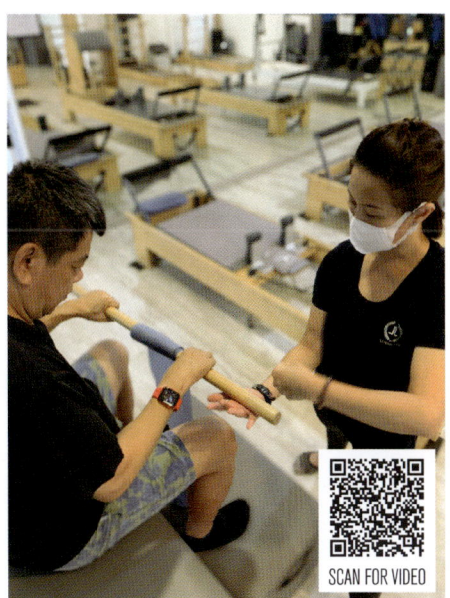

SCAN FOR VIDEO

Every session is a trial and error, an exploration of what works best for Terence. Adapting and tailoring the exercises to suit his specific needs became the core of our approach. It was about empowering him, bit by bit, to realise the potential within himself. What I really appreciate about Terence is that his sense of humour and love of life remains intact despite the challenges he faced.

I guess the key is to really find what resonates with each individual. In my approach as a fitness instructor, I have taken this to heart, striving to infuse every class I teach with elements of joy and playfulness. And in the midst of my busy routine, I do carve out moments to dance to a different tune, one being including my own kids in sessions of "Just Dance". Witnessing the young ones' genuine enjoyment and being able to instil an active lifestyle in them adds an extra layer of joy to my own happiness.

It is in these moments that I envision a promising future generation, one that values movement and health. As a parent and a fitness enthusiast, this vision motivates me to keep pushing forward, both in my personal fitness journey and in my role as a guide for others.

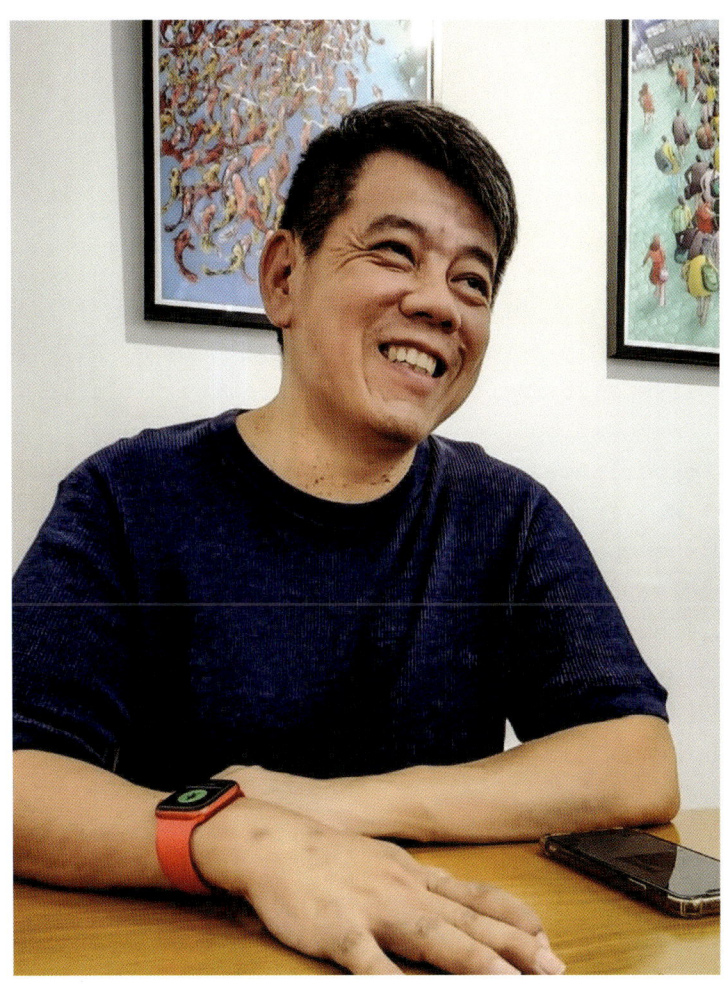

For years, I had dreamt of such a day. A day where I could wake up and not feel the fog in my mind, the weight of exhaustion on my shoulders. A day without the persistent reminders of physical and cognitive challenges. There was nothing more I wanted than to be free from the struggles that came with my stroke.

Yet, as I have discovered, the pursuit of such a day can overshadow the beauty found in the imperfect ones. The days where progress might be slow, but it is still progress.

Thinking back on my journey, stroke has certainly permeated every aspect of my life. But in its ironic generosity, it also bestowed upon me a wealth of lessons and experiences. The first of which is that it is overwhelming to constantly chase after the "perfect" day. In reality, there will always be the good, the bad, and the ugly. Focusing on making each day better than the previous one is a more attainable and fulfilling goal.

I remember the first few months after my stroke, where any form of movement felt like a Herculean task. But with each passing day, I pushed through the pain, and slowly, I saw progress. It was not always a straight line towards recovery, and there were plenty of setbacks and moments of frustration. Yet, through it all, I have grown stronger and more resilient.

This I have learnt, failure is certain. But it is not the end of the world; it is part and parcel of it. Failure teaches you more than success perhaps ever will. It toughens you up, forces you to reevaluate, and sometimes, is the kick in the ass you need to push yourself harder. These are the days that build resilience and character, teaching us that it is okay not to have it all together as long as we are still moving forward, bit by bit.

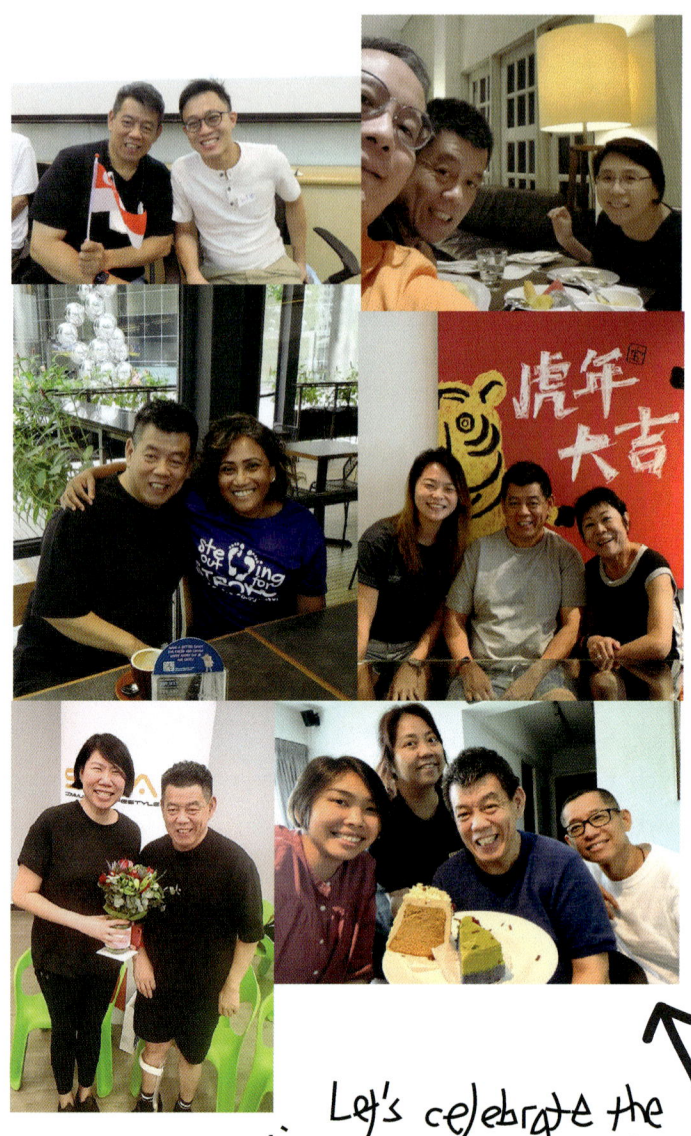

Let's celebrate the tiny joys that make life extraordinary! leaving the past in the rearview mirror and carving new paths ahead.

When life presents its inevitable trials, it is easy to succumb to despair. In cultivating gratitude, I've discovered that it is not just reserved for grand gestures or momentous occasions. It is in the everyday moments — the little thank yous to a stranger who holds the door open, the silent appreciation for a star-studded night sky — where gratitude finds its truest expression.

Gratitude reminds me to be thankful for the medical professionals who have helped me heal and regain my life, as well as my friends and loved ones for always being there during the toughest moments. Their presence is a constant reassurance, a reminder that I am not alone in this fight.

Writing these books became my way of giving back and extending a hand to those who might be facing their own battles. In sharing my story, I hope that no one has to feel isolated in their struggles. If my words can resonate with just one person, letting them know they are not alone, then the purpose of putting pen to paper is fulfilled.

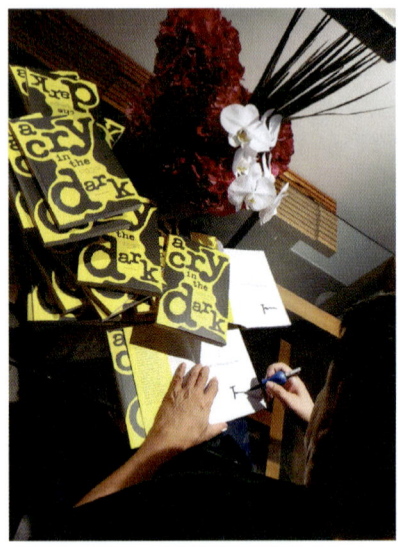

Sharing the real, the messy and the beautiful, because every chapter has its own story to tell ～

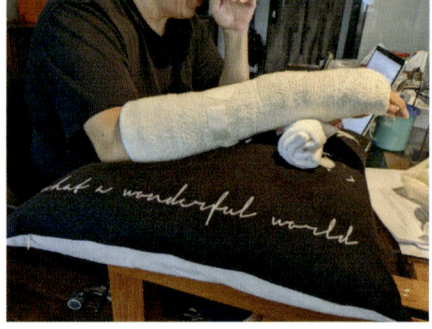

I have seen firsthand how the solace and understanding found in the experiences of others can be a powerful source of comfort. And really, it is the lens through which we view our circumstances that greatly influences our ability to overcome them. It is not said enough, but a positive outlook can make a world of a difference.

The road ahead may wind and twist, but armed with the lessons of the past, the support of my community, and the companionship of those who have walked this path beside me, I step into the future with a heart full of hope. I know that together, we can continue to defy the odds, one step at a time.

As I turn the pages of this chapter, I do
so with a heart filled with gratitude.
Gratitude for the challenges that sculpted
my character and the friendships that
blossomed in adversity. And gratitude for
the stroke that may have rewritten the
script of my life, but also opened my eyes
to a new and brighter future.

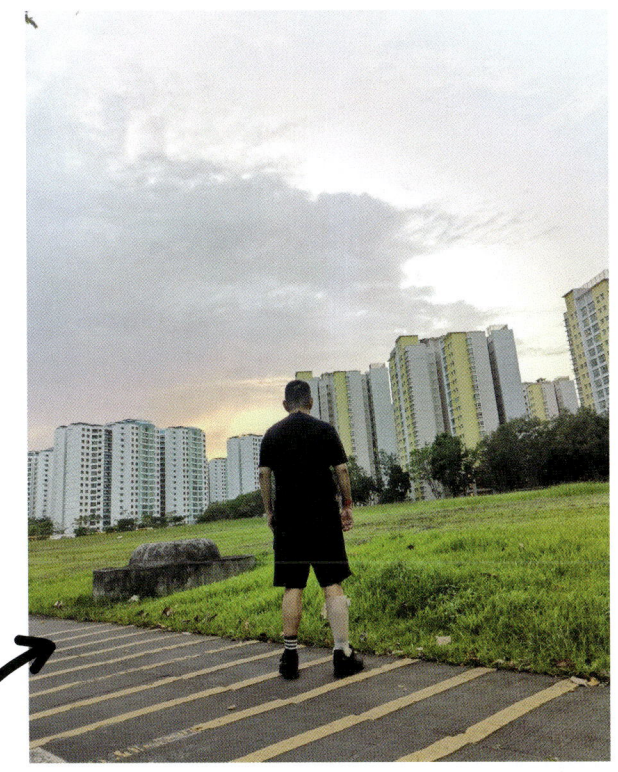

Each heartbeat is a precious gift, a
reminder that I am alive and kicking-
and to make it count!

"Having a stroke doesn't make me any less. I can still do whatever regular folks do."

— Ng Shu Kun

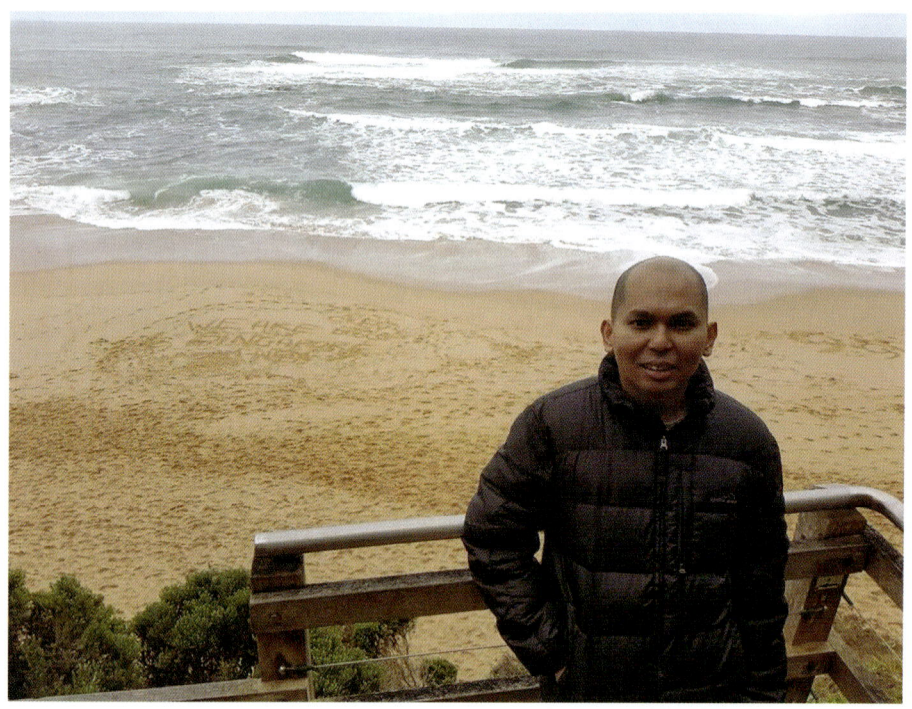

The year was 2010. I was stationed in Idaho, pulling my weight as an engineer in the Republic of Singapore Air Force (RSAF), happily married, and enjoying a typical night out with friends. Little did I know, life had an unexpected twist waiting for me.

As I got back home, I suddenly felt dizzy and collapsed. At first, I thought it was just a hangover, but as things worsened, I realised something was seriously wrong. My left side had clocked out, and there was slurring when I tried to speak.

My wife, a nurse, suspected stroke symptoms and wasted no time rushing me to a medical centre. Unfortunately, they lacked the facilities to treat a stroke, so I was airlifted to a state emergency care centre. The delay was excruciating, but eventually, the diagnosis came: Moyamoya disease, a rare condition causing blood vessel narrowing and blockage to the brain.

In a state of disbelief, I questioned why this happened. I had a comprehensive health check, and everything seemed fine. But some things cannot be predicted or explained. The damage was done. If treated during the golden period, I could have fully recovered, but that ship had sailed.

Moyamoya disease is a progressive illness, and I was told the only option was brain bypass surgery. Genetic factors seemed to play a role, adding to the frustration. But miraculously, within a day, I could walk again, though my left side still lacked control. After being hospitalised for three weeks, I was discharged.

I was to return to Singapore, where Moyamoya treatment was available. Physiotherapy in the United States (US) followed for a month or two, and my wife handled the logistics in the midst of the chaos — settling the car, apartment, and everything else. The RSAF was supportive, even flying my mom over. Due to the high risk of relapse during air travel, a medical team was also dispatched to ensure my safe journey home.

Back in Singapore, more tests at the National University Hospital (NUH) revealed no need for surgery yet. Annual check-ups that followed also showed positive indicators, and daily medication, physiotherapy, and acupuncture gradually improved my condition.

Doctors told me running was impossible, but something deep within me refused to accept that fate. I remembered the rush of endorphins and sense of accomplishment after pushing myself to new limits. And so, despite the doubts and fears of others, I decided to try.

Little by little, my overall gait improved. I regained more sensation in my limbs and could run longer distances without stopping. I even participated in the OCBC Cycle a few times. Each time I crossed the finish line of a race, it brought me back to life. I knew that anything was possible if you were willing to fight for it.

Despite the adjustments brought about by my condition, I managed to maintain a commendable performance in RSAF. Although no longer on the front lines, I took on a role behind the scenes, working on F15s. My body might have been limited, but my mind and spirit were not. In my new role at headquarters, what mattered most was my ability to contribute meaningfully in other ways.

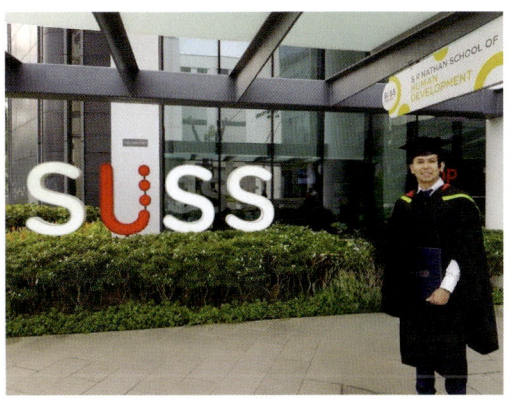

In 2014, I embarked on a degree in aerospace engineering. This would later shape my professional endeavours as I decided to pursue a career switch to IT,

particularly within the field of cloud computing at ST Engineering. Alongside my professional pursuits, I even managed to start a family, although concerns do linger about passing on symptoms to my child.

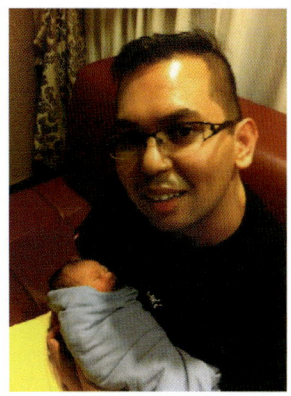

Reflecting on my journey so far, I realised
that nothing I had done was ever a waste.
Every obstacle, setback and challenge
helped shape me into the person I am today.
It may have been difficult at times to
see beyond the struggles, but I can now
understand how each experience contributed
to my growth. This new perspective gives me
the strength to keep moving forward, even
when things seem impossible.

"Recovery can be fun if you put some creativity into it."

— Atika Ahmad

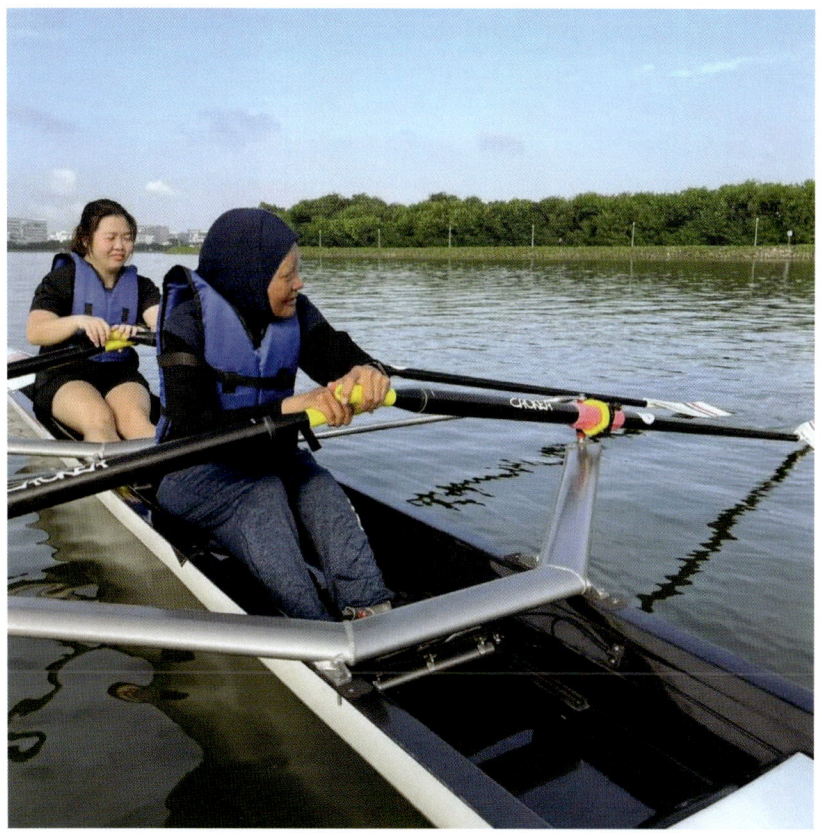

Looking back, it is hard to believe how much my life has changed in just a few years. From working in a canteen to surviving a stroke to setting up a home baking business, it has been a long and challenging journey.

It all started with my mom fighting stage 4 cancer in 2018, a battle she sadly lost in 2019. Her passing left a great impact on me, and I decided not to go back to working in the canteen but choose a different path for myself. As fate would have it, I was about to face my own health challenges.

2021 was the year I had my stroke. I remember waking up in the early hours of the morning, unable to stand or make my way to the bathroom. It was terrifying, but perhaps out of denial, I just brushed it off. When similar symptoms occurred the next day, my sister, drawing from past experiences, insisted I seek medical help.

The journey to the hospital was swift: they pushed me past the triage and straight to the doctor, highlighting the urgency of the situation. It turned out to be a blood clot on the right brain, impacting the left side of my body.

I was hospitalised after, and visits became solitary affairs as everyone tried to navigate the conditions of the COVID-19 pandemic. I had a lot of time to reflect on my life; the realisation that this was indeed a stroke eventually sank in. Research led me to support groups — it was a lifeline, just as it had been during my mother's cancer battle.

In particular, the support of the Singapore National Stroke Association (SNSA) brought a befriender, Sow Wei, into my life. His help was invaluable, guiding me and providing motivation to face the difficulties ahead. I was determined to give it my all and make full use of the golden period of recovery.

Physiotherapy and occupational therapy became part of my routine. The restrictions of the pandemic also forced a transition to online fitness groups, but I participated in these home workouts whenever I could. A mini pilgrimage, virtual Stepping Out for Stroke, and meetings — when the restrictions were lifted — with my workout buddies at Changi Village became like mini milestones for me.

From tying my hair to buttoning my shirt, every small accomplishment was something I held onto dearly. The support of non-stroke friends who just wanted to exercise together was also an unexpected but welcome surprise. And my sister, who has been there for me all along, got me to join her in her home baking business, putting back purpose and work in my life.

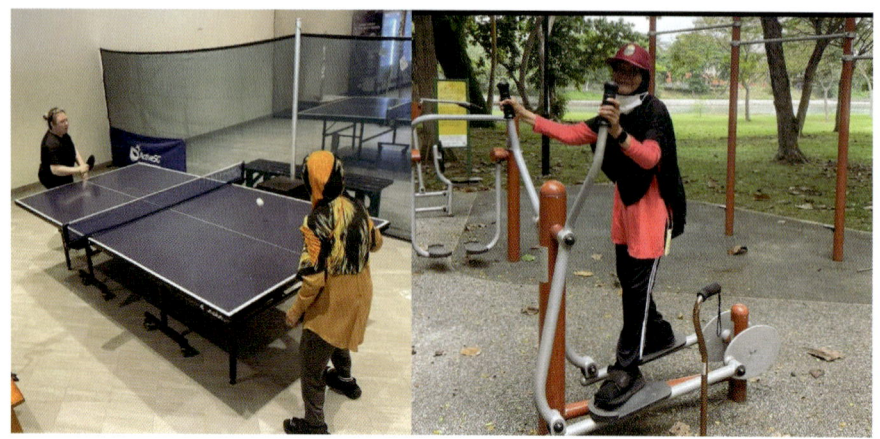

A year into recovery, my life has become more vibrant and active. While I used to be inactive and had little interest in sports, now I cannot get enough of it. From exploring interesting places to listening to music during workouts, I have found creative ways to keep the journey fun for me. I even picked up rowing, which has become like a source of freedom.

Through this journey, I have learned that although therapy can be expensive, taking charge of your own life does not have to be. I realised that I do not need to buy fancy workout equipment to exercise; I can simply be resourceful and find everyday objects around my home and neighbourhood that serve the same purpose. All it takes is determination, creativity, and finding joy in the journey. And with the support of friends and loved ones, anything is possible.

GRATEFUL STEPS

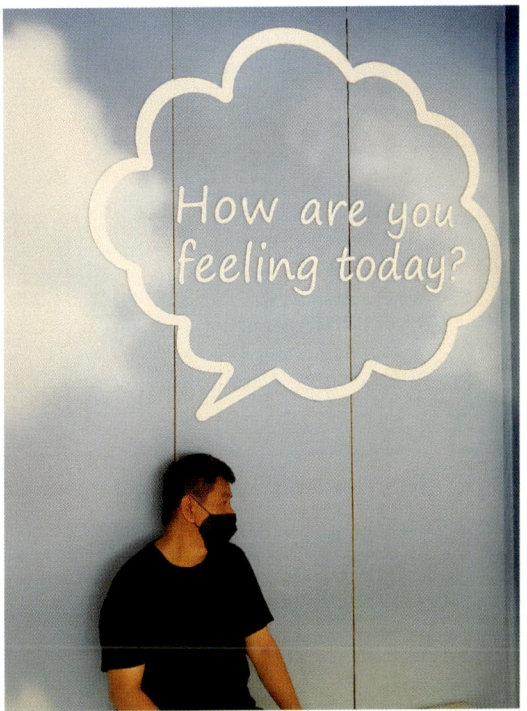

Strokes are often misunderstood, and it is time to change that. I, like many others, once believed it was an affliction of the elderly or those with pre-existing conditions. But the truth is, strokes can knock on anyone's door unexpectedly. They can affect anyone at any age, regardless of their health status.

Talking about strokes and sharing information is very important. Many people still do not know much about strokes and might have wrong ideas. Some people also believe that having a stroke is the end of a good life, which can be discouraging. Raising awareness helps break down this stigma and negative belief. It shows that life can still be fulfilling and meaningful after a stroke.

My own experience has taught me the importance of understanding the risk factors, recognising the symptoms and seeking prompt medical attention.

Early recognition and response are crucial. The "golden period of recovery" after a stroke is a window of opportunity, and time is of the essence. The quicker the medical intervention, the better the chances of minimising damage and achieving a more complete recovery. Recognising the signs and symptoms of a stroke and knowing to call for help without delay can be a life-saving decision.

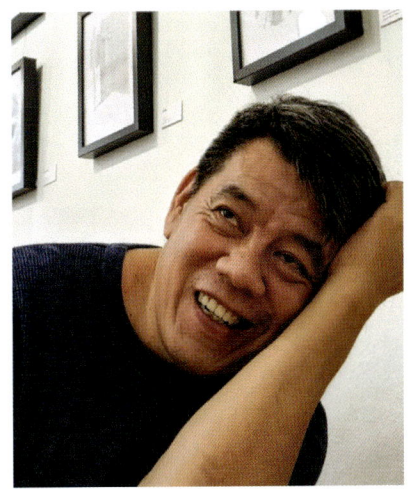

Every stroke is unique, and as a result, the challenges we face can be very diverse. Among the many physical, cognitive and emotional struggles we face, we must also navigate a new normal. The life we once knew transforms drastically, and the changes can be mentally and emotionally taxing.

The more people understand about strokes, the better prepared they can be to respond and seek the help they may need. For caregivers, communication is key. Talk to the survivor about their experience and their needs. Everyone's journey is unique, and tailoring support to individual circumstances is vital. Understand that recovery is a process, and it can be slow and unpredictable. Be patient with your loved one as they navigate their challenges.

Showing the world the new me was the best way to honour my resilience and the support I have received.

But at the same time, remember that taking care of yourself is not selfish. If you are supporting a loved one through stroke recovery, remember that you cannot pour from an empty cup. Seek support from stroke support groups, counselling, or healthcare professionals. You do not have to go through this journey alone.

When it comes to supporting stroke survivors, empathy plays a pivotal role. As friends, family, and community members, it is essential that we educate ourselves about these challenges to offer the right kind of support that truly makes a difference. This includes promoting accessibility in public spaces, advocating for workplace accommodations, and fostering a culture of inclusion.

It requires ongoing education and a commitment to addressing the multifaceted challenges stroke survivors face. By cultivating awareness, providing practical assistance, and fostering emotional support, we can significantly contribute to the well-being and quality of life of those on their journey to recovery.

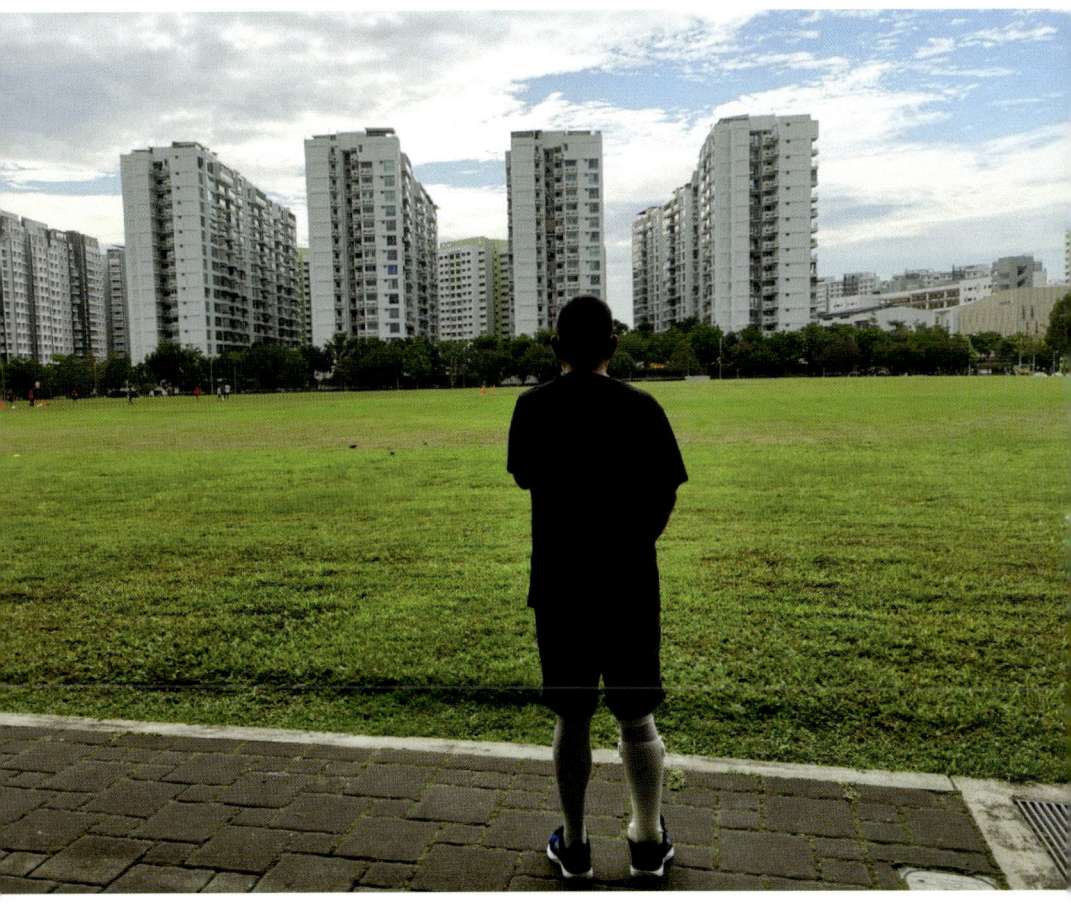

Encouraged by the tremendous success of his first two books, *Emerging from the Dark* and *A Cry in the Dark*, Terence is yet again gifting us with his latest book on exercise, *Strength in Motion*.

Terence has successfully overcome many challenges experienced by a stroke survivor, such as cognitive impairment, emotional and psychosocial difficulties, and social isolation. He did this with much grit and determination.

All of us who desire to stay fit know what it takes — a regime of proper diet and exercise. Many of us were enthusiastic enough to purchase stationary bikes, cross-trainers, treadmills, and rowing machines. Truth is, many of these ended up in the heap of "white elephants" sitting pretty and unused because we lack the discipline to follow through.

That is why for yet another reason, Terence is an inspiring model. For him to have strength enough to keep moving and moving enough to gain strength after a severe stroke requires extraordinary discipline. This book can teach us more than a thing or two.

We need to help put this into the hands of every stroke survivor and encourage them to read it. This book will inspire and impact them to work towards recovery the way Terence recovered.

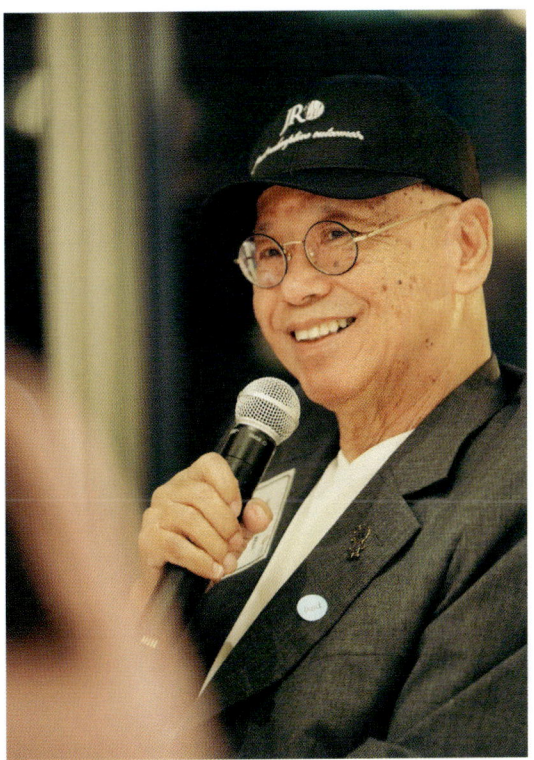

DR. WILLIAM WAN, JP, PHD

SENIOR CONSULTANT, SINGAPORE KINDNESS MOVEMENT

Strength in Motion is Terence Ang's third book, following *A Cry in the Dark* and *Emerging from the Dark*.

Terence has a natural flair for writing and is able to give a detailed and positive account of his recovery from a petrifying stroke that left him paralysed and unable to speak. His personality also shines through in his books, showing his friendly, caring nature.

The challenges he faced adjusting to his new life — receiving regular physiotherapy, occupational and speech therapy — are vividly portrayed in this new book. It is a complex endurance journey with many peaks and valleys, but Terence is someone who has the tenacity to keep on going.

This book provides inspiration and hope for others, especially those facing similar challenges. I can highly recommend it.

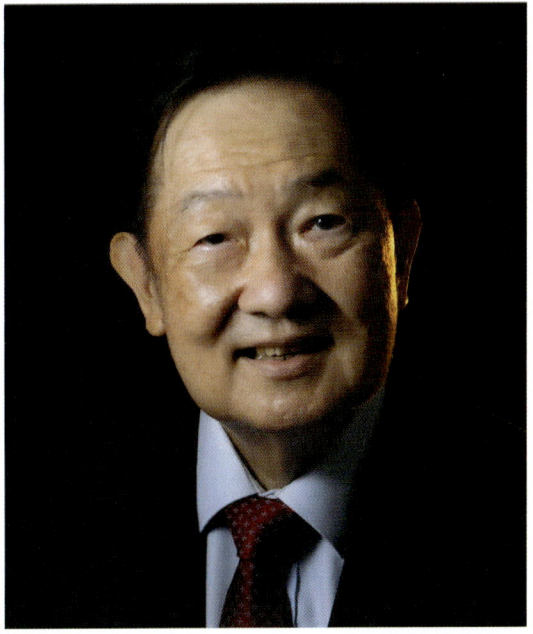

DR. KENNETH LYEN

Dr. Kenneth Lyen is a consultant paediatrician in Singapore and founder of the Rainbow Centre for children with disabilities and those on the autism spectrum. He is also a composer of musical theatre and author of books and articles, having published 16 books on the mental health of children and other topics.

Before his stroke, Terence was known for his marketing prowess, transforming brands and companies that he worked with. Post-stroke, Terence has taken that talent and turned it inward into a journey of resilience, transforming himself and his personal story into inspiration for stroke survivors and their caregivers everywhere. We don't always have a say in the cards that life deals us, but we definitely can choose how we want to play those cards. Get ready, because Terence is about to bring the house down!

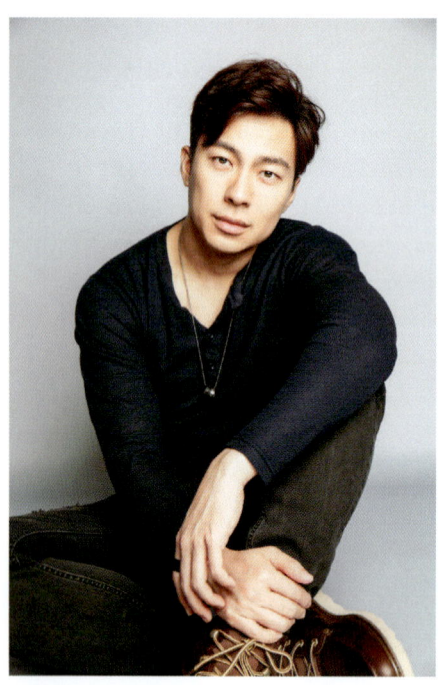

NAT HO

*ACTOR, SINGER,
SONGWRITER,
ENTREPRENEUR*

Terence's life is truly a beacon of hope for those facing similar challenges. Through his books, he continues to inspire and uplift, showing that with faith and determination, one can weather any storm and emerge stronger than ever. I have had the privilege of working with Terence, and I have always respected his creativity and trailblazing attitude. I will forever be thankful for his involvement in my first movie, *Perfect Rivals*, as it received much media coverage with his involvement. Seeing his book illuminate NYC Times Square as an Amazon Bestseller is nothing short of extraordinary. I am so proud of him. Big hugs and congratulations on your success, Dear!

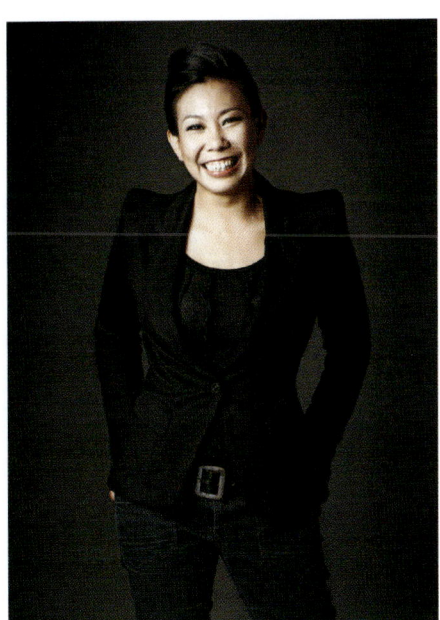

IRENE ANG

FOUNDER & CEO OF
FLY ENTERTAINMENT

ACKNOWLEDGEMENTS

Editor-in-chief
Mickey Hiah

Special thanks to all who have generously
shared their stories and insights, and greatly
enriched this book (in order of appearance):

Assoc. Prof. Gan Wee Hoe, Dr. Wee Tze Chao,
Dr. Shamala Thilarajah, Evelyn Khoo, Lim Hai
Yen, Sijie Lin, Tan Kha Seng, Joey Lee, Alvin
Chee, Koh Yan Fen, Dr. Moses Koh, Ann Ho, Ng
Shu Kun, Atika Ahmad, Dr. William Wan, Dr.
Kenneth Lyen, Nat Ho, Irene Ang

And to my family — James, Angela and Yew Teck
for always standing by me, without whom none
of this would have been possible.

Published by
World Scientific Publishing Co. Pte. Ltd.
5 Toh Tuck Link, Singapore 596224
USA office: 27 Warren Street, Suite 401-402, Hackensack, NJ 07601
UK office: 57 Shelton Street, Covent Garden, London WC2H 9HE

ISBN 978-981-12-9152-4 (hardcover)
ISBN 978-981-12-9170-8 (paperback)
ISBN 978-981-12-9153-1 (ebook for institutions)
ISBN 978-981-12-9154-8 (ebook for individuals)

For any available supplementary material, please visit
https://www.worldscientific.com/worldscibooks/10.1142/13795#t=suppl